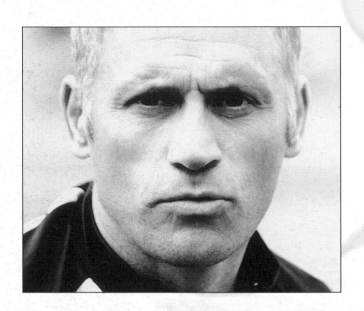

INSPIRED

the blueprint for total conditioning
Bernie Shrosbree

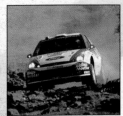

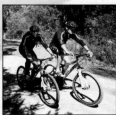

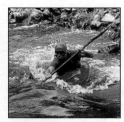

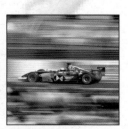

focus   **determination**   **no limits**   **performance**

For the ultimate team: my wife Kim and my son and daughter Gregg and Danielle.

Why Inspired? Well, the inspiration for writing this book, and in fact my whole way of life, has come from the amazing people I have met, worked with, learnt from and, most importantly, been inspired by.

Looking back, I would single out Rick Grice who spotted something in me at the tender age of 13; if the timing's right, it's amazing how much someone's influence can stay with you for the rest of your life. Rick gave me a huge insight into what a life dedicated to sport could be about and, to this day, I still have the same passion for challenging the outdoors that he inspired over thirty years ago. Rick died on 6th August 1986 during an attempt on Mont Blanc and I hope he's up there somewhere watching me still doing it…

Finally, a big thanks (and much respect) to all of you out there who, over the years, have helped me in my sports career – your coaching and support has meant that I have gone a long way towards reaching my potential as a sportsman. Too many to name, but you know who you are.

Bernie Shrosbree
July 2004

Contents

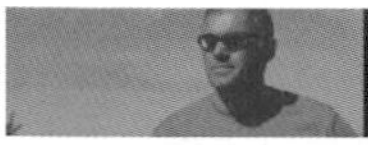

Being inspired   6

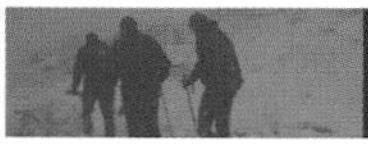

Shrosbree's six of the best   24

Running and walking **26**; Progression in your training **38**; Cycling **42**; Swimming **54**; Kayaking **62**; Rowing **68**; Cross-country skiing **74**

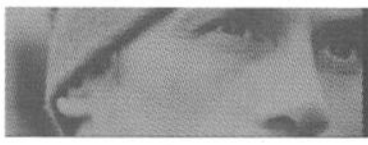

Where are you now?   80

Heart rate monitors **86**

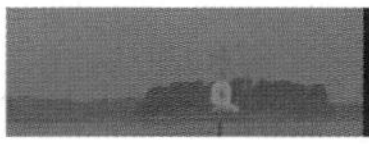

Basic conditioning   90

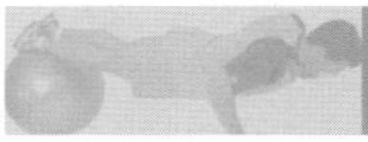

Core stability and functional training   104

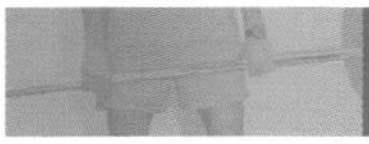

Compound exercises   114

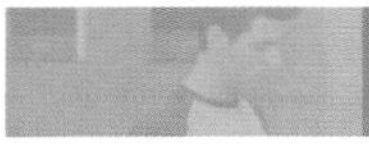

The muscle groups   126

The shoulders **128**; The upper back **138**; The chest **154**; The arms **164**; The trunk and lower back **176**; The legs **190**

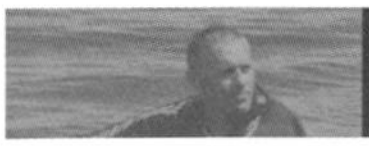

Warm-up, cool down and stretching   204

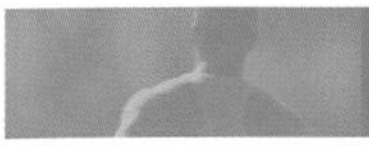

Enjoying the environment   218

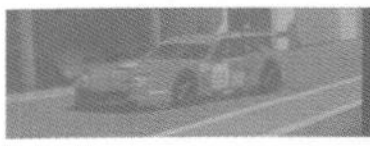

Mind games   230

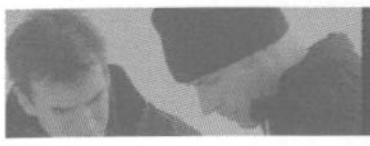

Programme planning   238

Index   253

Foreword

by James Cracknell

THE FIRST TIME I MET BERNIE Shrosbree was during a warm weather training camp in Lanzarote. Bernie happened to be at the same location working with three Formula One drivers – Jenson Button, Mark Webber and Giancarlo Fisichella – and he came over to help us with some cycling sessions.

I was immediately drawn to this character who always gives 100% and has massive enthusiasm for sport in general, which makes it easy to follow his lead – and that's even before you know anything about him. Then you find out how many different sports Bernie has excelled in (although he's the last person to boast about them) and you start understanding his philosophy of 'you can enjoy sports and do them properly', which is a refreshing approach because quite a lot of our training is basically 'do it hard, get it done'.

For example, on those cycling sessions in Lanzarote, Bernie was very keen to show us how to cycle with good technique. He didn't want us to train hard while riding badly or cycle just for the sake of getting fit. He had exactly the same attitude when he took us skiing some time later: yes, get fit from the skiing, but also enjoy it as a sport.

Bernie has been a massive influence on our cross-country skiing camps. Nothing is too much effort in whatever he is doing. He'll go skiing in the morning, ski with us and then take people for extra skiing if they want to do that, as well as organising the camp. If you are enthusiastic and want to get stuck in he'll give you that extra edge, bit of attention and effort. All of which makes you very loyal to him: it wasn't surprising that when Jenson Button changed teams, he wanted Bernie to go with him.

Bernie is many things: he's done a huge variety of sports and served in the armed forces. Rather than say 'I've got a massive trophy cabinet' he says 'look at the experience I have'. To get the respect from sportsmen the way he does (including from some very picky Olympic gold medallists!) without a haul of world records is a testament to his character, who he is and how he does it: to have performed under intense pressure in the armed services, and reached international standard in two or three sports is very, very rare. But it's also less daunting because maybe people will think, 'perhaps I can do some of the things Bernie has done'.

It's good to see that Bernie has decided to explain his approach and his philosophy in this book – which is full of his personality and completely different from so many of the other, frankly boring, exercise and fitness books. If you can incorporate Bernie's approach to exercise into your life – even if you think you don't have any extra time available – you will be surprised at how much more energy you have for everything else. You may feel more tired at the outset, but you will soon see how your quality of life improves in terms of what you can achieve – without having to become a Lycra-clad sports geek.

I'm glad to see that he has put such a strong emphasis on the importance of core stability work, which we do a lot of so that the strength we have can be applied efficiently; and on setting achievable goals. It's vital that people have a goal in their training programme, whether it's with the aim of competing, doing it with mates or just a personal test on the rowing machine – that sense of aiming for a specific target makes it so much easier to train.

Bernie's enthusiasm is genuinely infectious and that comes across in this book, along with the almost instinctive understanding of what is important in body conditioning, all of which is based on real experience.

Enjoy getting to know Bernie in the coming pages: and take my advice – take his advice!

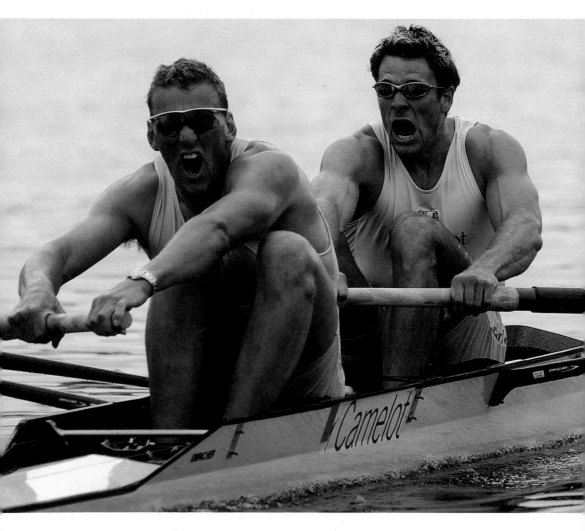

How hard is hard? Pinsent and Cracknell push it to the limit

Being inspired

THIS BOOK IS ACTUALLY MEANT TO BE about you rather than about me, because I want it to help you achieve your full potential. But I do want to tell you something about myself and my experience, simply because it will help you to understand what has motivated me and where my particular brand of thinking about performance and training comes from.

Some people call this my 'philosophy', but that's far too fancy a word for what it is. I just happen to have a particular way of looking at the whole business of conditioning, exercise and training. And that comes from two things: my own personal experience, and the people who helped me gain that experience. Although I've never thought that I'm the world's greatest athlete, and I'm not a sports science graduate (although luckily for me I work with people who are both of those things), I do have a background that is not that common: I've been an international athlete in two very different disciplines – winter biathlon and triathlon – and I served both as a Royal Marine and as a special forces soldier in the SBS – the Special Boat Squadron – all of which taught me a certain kind of attitude.

But even before I got involved in sports and before I joined the Marines, I was learning from good people who taught me about dedication, commitment and enthusiasm. From being somebody who had a certain amount of insecurity and a lack of confidence (probably true of most of us), I was shown a way to achieve success in sport, not as a show-off or a smartarse, but in a way that meant I actually enjoyed the whole experience.

When I was a kid I have to admit I was a bit of a tearaway. I had far too much energy and absolutely no discipline. For some kids, having so much energy – being hyperactive, in other words – could have led to problems, especially if I hadn't had any positive route for soaking it all up. But I was lucky. I had a number of influential and inspirational role models at critical points in my life who taught me a different way of using all that energy, of channelling it for a specific purpose, and who showed me how I could get a buzz from taking part in challenging sports that kept me fit and healthy.

Thanks to their encouragement and advice, by the time I was 18 I was representing my country as an international athlete, by the age of 25 I was challenging to become champion of *Survival of the Fittest* in the UK, and at 30 I was runner-up in the World *Survival of the Fittest*.

These other people, these role models – coaches, trainers, mentors and friends – have been my personal inspiration. In this book I want to share some of their advice with you as well as passing on my own thoughts and ideas, so that you can have as much fun as I have over the years, and

'Because you're worth it!'

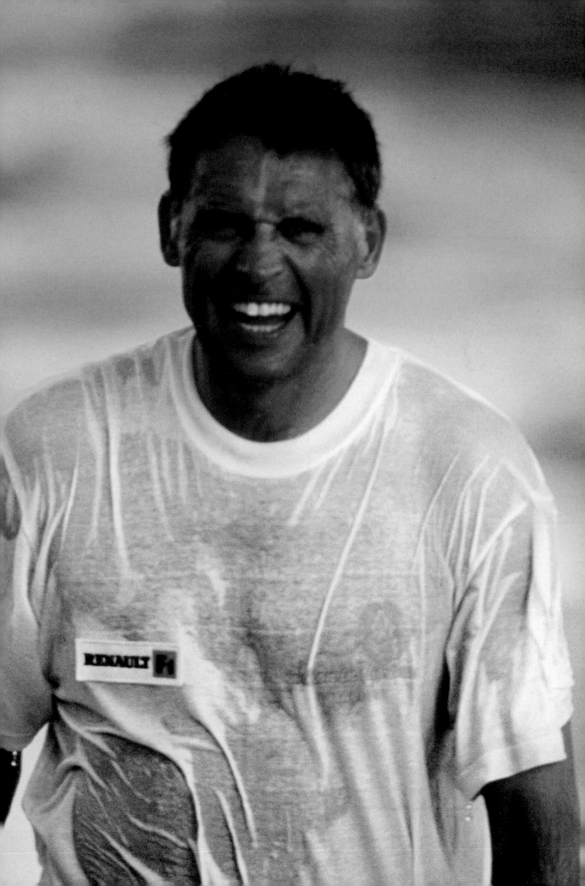

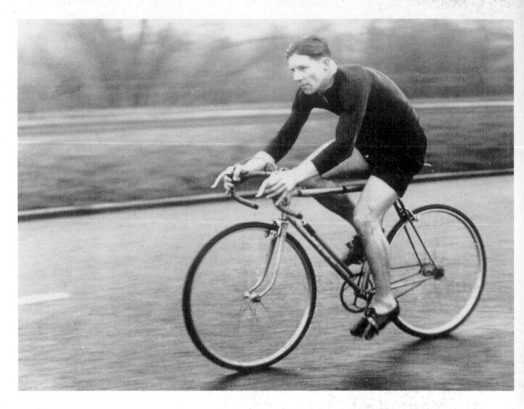

turn that into inspiration for increasing your fitness to the level you would like it to be through a better sporting performance. If we can achieve that together, we'll both be happy.

Because I always try to draw on my own experience, I want to tell you a little bit about my story. So bear with me for a few pages and then we'll get onto the really important subject of this book – you.

My earliest memory of sports and fitness is of a time when I was about 8. My brother Paul was four years older than me and a member of the Hornchurch Harriers Athletics Club. He was running in a 800 metre race (it was 880 yards back then) and I remember being on the outside of the track and running alongside the competitors. I think I managed to stay with them for a couple of hundred metres before these older boys left me behind.

What made me do that? My parents

hadn't said, "Go and race". I had simply become caught up in the excitement of seeing my brother competing and wanted to be part of the challenge. I still do. Whenever there's some sport on TV I really struggle to watch it unless I can concentrate on gaining some extra knowledge from somebody's technique. I'd much rather be out there taking part.

Paul is now a father of two who still enjoys jogging and playing football. Forty-odd years ago he was good at organising off-the-cuff races in the neighbourhood where we grew up, at Rainham in Essex. We'd get a bunch of our cousins and friends together and have competitions racing round the terraced houses. That was one way I could try to emulate the runners I watched at the Hornchurch Harriers (which is now known as Havering AC).

Before they'd had us kids, my parents

Charlie Shrosbree, my dad, competing in a 25-mile time trial in 1952

Remember, there's always a reason not to do something. This book is about reminding yourself of the reasons you really want to do it.

had been actively involved in the Leo Cycling Club in Essex, and had both reached a good competitive club standard. Even though my father didn't have as much time for sport when I was growing up, he still managed to keep fit. He was a welder at the Ford car factory – every day he'd cycle into work, and at weekends he'd pop out for the odd ride or for a quick run.

Sometimes I'd be taken along too for a run in the nearby park. If we were going to Hainault Forest, I wouldn't be able to sleep because I was so excited about escaping out of the built-up area where we lived and exploring the lanes of the forest on a bike or running with my dad for a couple of hours. I was so keen to get into that environment, and so naturally active, that sometimes I'd just head off from home and run in the forest for hours on end.

One time, when I was five years old and we were on holiday at East Wittering in Sussex, I started running along the beach all the way to West Wittering. I got lost and the police took me to the local station so that my parents could come and collect me. I was so exhausted that I fell straight to sleep as soon as I got inside the police station.

All this energy meant that I spent a lot of time being frustrated, especially at school where it seemed as if the only thing I was able to concentrate on was the bell which marked the end of each lesson so that I could get outside and play.

My personal breakthrough came when I was about 12 or 13. Two of the teachers at my school used to take groups canoeing on a lake – actually more like a big pond – in the countryside ten miles or so away. The moment I sat in a canoe all that random energy I possessed suddenly became entirely focused. I knew then that I wanted to be involved in a sport which took me out into the great environment of rivers, trees, rocky mountains and coastlines.

Although I'm sure I would not have been able to articulate the thought at the time, I realised that here was a way that I could release my natural energy through some kind of organised physical activity. It was an amazing feeling after so much pent-up frustration. I would spend hours and hours concentrating on mastering the technique of canoeing up to a level that I thought was perfection … If only I'd felt the same way about studying, I could have been a top scientist by now!

That's why the outdoor environment has always played such an important part in my life. There is nothing quite like the buzz you get after a hard run in the mountains, surrounded by the glories of nature – with the smell of the pines and the granite rock making you feel good anyway – then stopping at the top of a climb, after all that hard work, and taking time to look at and respond to the natural world. Or when, in the mists of the early morning, out on the river for a paddle with some friends in our kayaks, we marvel at the breathtakingly beautiful scenery. You might think that words like 'glorious', 'beautiful' and 'nature' seem odd in a book about fitness. Don't believe it – they're part and parcel of the inspiration.

For me, paddling on the river in the

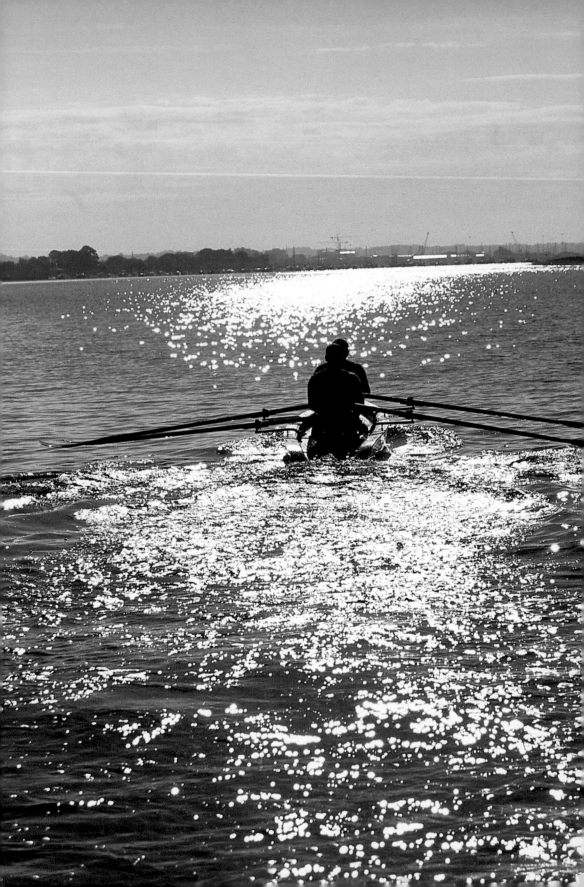

An early morning row in Poole harbour
Rick Grice climbing in the 1970s. Rick was a very good mountaineer who tragically died
during an attempt on Mont Blanc. It was Rick who inspired me to get out there at five
o'clock in the morning to swim, run and canoe. I've followed his way ever since

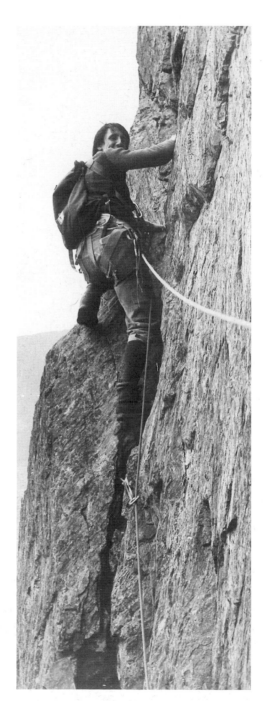

early morning mist with nobody else around is totally inspiring, with the herons flying past to salute my efforts and the kingfishers darting in and out of their riverbank nests in support of my achievement. That's exactly how I like it, quite selfish, really: I like to be alone. It's like the moment in cross-country skiing when you leave a marked trail in a Norwegian forest and head out onto virgin snow: that sense that you are the only person who has ever been there.

With my new-found sense of purpose I started, for the first time in my life, to want to achieve things. My parents sent me on an Outward Bound course at Holme Park in Devon where we were put into teams, or 'watches', and did a whole range of activities including orienteering, white water canoeing, climbing, rafting and navigation. By the end of the course I had been awarded the prize for the most outstanding performer. I had also learnt an obvious but important lesson: that being surrounded by great colleagues and quality coaches can bring out the best in you.

One of the first people to help me was a guy called Rick Grice, who was the head of outdoor pursuits for the Havering educational authorities. Rick was an excellent canoeist and mountaineer. Of course I looked up to him immensely, because he was doing the things I wanted to do, and doing them extremely well. Rick amazingly (or astutely, take your pick!) spotted some kind of basic talent in me, and encouraged me to work hard. I was so enthused about kayaking, for example, that I thought nothing of jumping on a bike and cycling ten miles to sit and paddle for an hour before cycling all the way home again. At school I tried to do as many sports as I could, whether it was basketball or pole vaulting. Most nights I was completely exhausted.

All that activity was fine, but I still needed to find some kind of context for it. As I came to the end of my school days I had to go out and earn money. At the time no career path for sports scientists or trainers existed, so it never crossed my mind as an option. Instead I went to work in a local supermarket. I had never been so unhappy and knew I could not carry on working there. I did think about teaching canoeing but again there was no established way to go about that. So I joined the Royal Marines.

To this day, I say that they stitched me up ... I saw a photo in a Marines brochure of special forces soldiers paddling canoes and thought, 'I'd like to do that.' The soldiering aspect was not of any great interest. I went into a recruiting centre and before I knew it the Marines sergeant had persuaded me to sign on the dotted line (the date is drilled into my memory – it was 4th November 1975), my head was shaved, and it was 'Welcome to the Marines.' Two years later I realised I still hadn't seen a single bloody canoe!

In fact, I have a lot to thank the Royal Marines for. Their training course was full of physical challenges and to get through it you had to learn incredible discipline. The energy I had had all through my early teens was still pretty untamed when I joined the Marines, but by the time I got my green beret, I had come to see that brute force and ignorance didn't achieve much; it was mental discipline, controlled energy and teamwork that could work wonders. It was a great honour to complete the course because I knew I'd be working with a great unit of men.

After the passing-out parade, I joined 45 Commando in Arbroath, Scotland. This was my dream job, specialising in arctic and mountain warfare. A lot of our time was spent training on the Isle of Skye, up on the Cuillin Ridge, in an incredible environment. In the winter of 1977 we went over to Norway for three months of arctic warfare training at Moriana. This was all about learning how to survive in snowholes at temperatures of −40ºC – or worse. If you were not properly prepared you just would not survive the night; and more importantly you were only as good as your team. There was no room for drama queens or big egos.

On that trip I had my first taste of cross-country skiing, of skiing full stop. At the end of the training course there was a 20km biathlon race. At one point I was leading by five clear minutes, loving the grace of sliding through the snow tracks between the pine trees in this magical white landscape. It was overwhelming. So overwhelming, in fact, that I promptly collapsed, got picked up by a snow vehicle and was carted off to the sick bay.

But again, as with Rick Grice, somebody had identified that maybe, just maybe, I could work on some raw, basic skills. This was Corporal Neil Bowman, who was running the Royal Marines' Nordic ski biathlon team; every year he would add two junior Marines to the team and train them to represent the corps at the Junior British Biathlon and

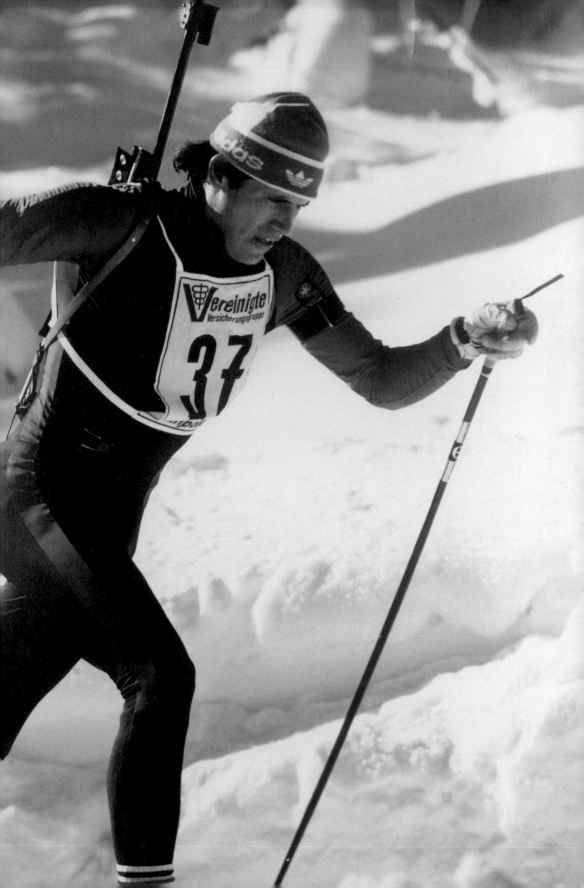

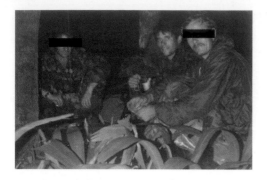

Jungle warfare training – another example of team-work and discipline

Nordic Ski Championships. Neil is a quiet guy, with a laid-back but very disciplined coaching attitude. The impact of that attitude on me was both immediate and exciting. At 18, in my first season, I found myself taking part in the Interservices Cross-Country Ski Championships, landing a top six place which led to a trial for the British team. For the Marines this was good PR, and I was given permission to train full time. In 1981, my third season, I was British Nordic ski champion.

I was very lucky to have been found by Neil, somebody who could understand the potential of my energies and who knew how to hone and channel them. He also taught me the importance of technique, that there was no point in thrashing away on skis as hard as possible without having the right technique.

We would spend whole days gliding up and down a frozen lake learning and practising the principles of cross-country skiing, breaking it down into specific elements and concentrating on each one in turn. I was blessed with plenty of stamina and endurance (thanks to my parents), but that on its own wasn't enough. I also possessed a strong competitive streak, but that wasn't enough either. Neil's training and the emphasis on technique made all the difference.

The success that I was able to have in Nordic skiing led to an increase in my own confidence and consequently gave me a sharper mental edge. I knew that somebody else might be fitter than me, but I was now able to switch on an extra psychological element to fight to be a winner. Mentally I knew that I could achieve something special.

At the time, however, there was no real structure in the UK for cross-country skiing, certainly nothing that could even begin to compete with the Scandinavians and the Russians. And when I found myself in the national team, Neil Bowman was not involved – I really missed his input, his encouragement and his wisdom. Although I had some talent, I could not see how I was going to progress in that sport. It was time to move on.

In my professional career, I had the option to leave the Marines, but (still holding onto the image of the Marines canoeing that had inspired me to join in the first place) I decided to stick with it, and transferred onto the Special Boat Service course. I thought this would suit my particular interests and skills. It was the wake-up call from hell: a two-week 'acquaint course', as they called it, that basically acquainted you with a lot of pain. Out of the one hundred and twenty-five on the course, five – including one B. Shrosbree – passed. Only seven guys had passed from the previous course.

The course effectively lasted two years. Week in, week out, you were pushed and tested; sometimes you felt that it would never end. I clearly remember being stuck up in the mountains on one exercise and seeing a lighted window in a farmhouse through my night vision goggles. Behind that window, I thought, is normality –

When I was on the SBS training course the biggest lie I was ever told was that every day has a start and every day has an end.

or pretty much most people's idea of normality. Up in the mountains my new normality was being physically exhausted, short on sleep and food, wet, cold and uncomfortable. Seeing that lighted window almost made me want to jack it all in and get my head down in a good warm bed. But what kept me going was the support and teamwork of the guys around me.

The Marines training involved training for the jungle, the desert, mountain and arctic warfare, and diving (diving is a major part of the SBS work). Each of us on the course had a different fear to overcome. Some guys would have a phobia about being in the jungle, others hated the desert, and some were spooked by working in the dark. For me it was the diving. I had felt pretty confident about the diving phase, as I'd been a member of a sub-aqua club for a while, but I can't tell you the horrors of the first open-water night dive I did, and just how spooked

and scared I was. Well, I can try to tell you, but I'm not sure my powers of description will do it justice.

There I was in the middle of Portsmouth harbour, with no torch, no lights, using only touch to make headway, squeezing underneath the hull of a boat a couple of metres above the silt on the harbour floor. I had to overcome real feelings of panic. I was hyperventilating and using up my air supply far too fast. I was sorted out by my buddy, my diving partner, who sensed through the line connecting us that I was in trouble, and tugged on the rope to let me know I was not alone down there in the blackness, that he'd make sure I was going to be OK. And I managed to master my fear. Even now, twenty years later, I could go out and do that dive again, because I know I have done it, I understand how it works. I've learnt not to be frightened of fear, not to let worrying about what might happen paralyse me.

I also learnt about patience. Anyone

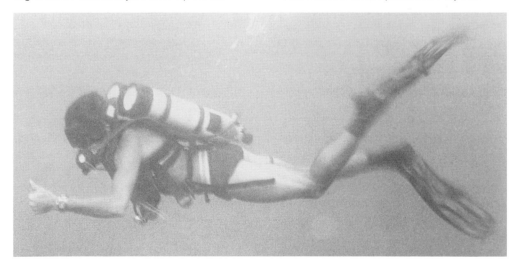

A pleasure dive with the SBS in the Blue Hole off the Keys in Belize

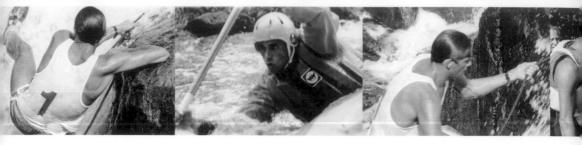

who knows me will tell you I'm a fidget; I find it difficult to sit still for very long. So imagine what it was like for me to have to lie in an observation post for a week hardly moving at all.

I learnt about surviving on the run after being dropped off with three other Marines in the middle of nowhere with no food, no money and no sleep, being chased round the south of England or the wilds of Scotland by a pack of police, service guys, dogs, choppers, the works – all taking a huge amount of pleasure in trying to prove we weren't up to the job. Not only did we have to evade that lot, but we also had to complete certain objectives and reach key points on an escape map on time.

It wasn't all total grimness. There was the time I managed to smuggle a fiver inside my shoe, and snuck myself in to (or 'inserted myself' in military jargon) a museum in a posh country house. It was tea time, and there I was smelling of the wet, rain and mud after a week in the field, in the tea queue with a coachload of grannies. When I got to the front of the queue, the only things available to buy (rather than the twenty Mars bars I'd had in mind), were four pieces of Black Forest gateau. When I got back to my teammates, there was nearly a lynching.

Another time, I was cooking dinner on a silt mudbank while another lad was working out the navigation. I dropped his dinner in the mud by accident, but deciding not to interrupt his very important map reading, I scooped up the meal, stuck it in his mess tin and passed it over to him. "Bit gritty", he remarked. He had the runs for a week.

In the SBS environment, they put you under pressure and then at the very moment you're feeling extreme fatigue, they say, 'Pack it in, you're not going to make it, Shrosbree' and tempt you with the thought of jacking it in, going back to camp for food and a nice warm shower. That was the most difficult part, because whereas I can handle an aggressive guy yelling in my face, it's the nice guy, the one who pretends he cares for you and offers you the chance to get warm and fed, who is the most dangerous – certainly as far as I am concerned.

We helped each other out, of course. I remember one canoeing exercise, a 30-mile paddle in the middle of winter, where the first thing they made us do was to capsize in the freezing waters; then we had to sit on the beach for an hour. I was desperate to get into the water and start paddling, but I could see one guy who was just sitting there, avoiding any eye contact, totally wrapped up in his own pain and about to lose it. That's when we rallied round to help, just like my Marine friend Pete Goss did when he made that decision in the middle of a raging storm to turn back and fight through 160 miles to help a fellow yachtsman, Raphael Dinelli, who was in difficulties.

You are drilled so well in the SBS

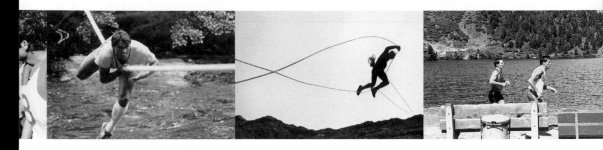

because they want you to feel that an actual operation is, well, if not exactly a walk in the park, then no worse than anything you've experienced during the training phase. So if you're diving from a submarine to get onto an oil rig in the North Sea or to board a warship under cover of darkness, you know that you can trust the sub commander, the guy opening the hatch to let you out and that the navigators have got the tides right – and that you can trust yourself to perform under these extreme conditions.

Sharing those difficult and gruelling times, in a deep, dark hole of physical, mental and emotional fatigue that, to be brutally honest, only a few of us have gone into, has created a brotherhood of men who will always support each other, even now they are out of the forces. Some of them, of course, find it very difficult to adjust to 'Civvy Street', and some never do, due to lack of trust.

Meanwhile, having moved on from Nordic skiing, I tried the challenge of the UK's *Survival of the Fittest* programme, an early 1980s TV foray into extreme sports such as they were at the time, which brought together a bunch of athletes from various disciplines, including fell runners, mountaineers, orienteers, potholers, cave divers – and me. Two events a day in the wet and the cold would be held over five consecutive days.

The organisers had approached Neil Bowman first, but he didn't think it was for him. However, he said he did know

one sucker who'd be perfect for what they had in mind, so they rang me.

The competition included a number of truly exhausting activities: the aerial ropes course was one of the most demanding things I've ever done in my life: the ideal competitor for that particular event would have been a jockey with arms like Arnold Schwarzenegger.

I asked the Marines instructors to give me some help in working on my upper body strength, and they took immense delight in coming up with innovative training sessions. In one exercise they strapped me into a climbing harness and attached the harness to the bars on the gym wall. Then they gave me a tug-of-war rope – at the other end of which were some burly Marines sitting on a gym mat. My job was to haul them towards me, while they showered me with friendly abuse. Believe me, don't try this one at home; it nearly ripped my arms out of their sockets. But it paid off.

I also spent time beforehand analysing each of the individual challenges, rather than ploughing in and hoping that brute force or fitness would get me through them. All of that preparation and pre-planning paid off. The guys who were superfit but had only ever done one main sport, and had trained for nothing else, found themselves struggling.

There were nine events in the first *Survival of the Fittest*, and I managed to win five and come second in the others. So there I was suddenly champion

The elements, the challenge, the buzz. Shrosbree at home in his natural environment – *Survival of the Fittest*, 1982

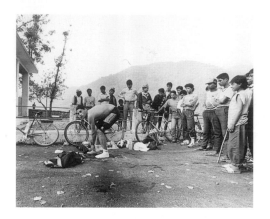

of *Survival of the Fittest* in 1982, and again for the next two years running. I think the organisers must have got bored with me, because they bunked me up to the *World Survival of the Fittest* finals, in which I got beaten by a superfit American guy, Dave Bingham, although in my defence I did smack a little too hard into the cliff face on the abseiling section. In any case, there was no danger of getting big-headed about any success I might have had, as I always had to go back to the Marines, who were highly trained in the fine art of bringing you right back down to earth.

All these activities came together when after a year in the SBS someone told me about a new sport called 'triathlon', which three US Seals – a Navy swimmer, a top cyclist and a marathon runner – had cooked up in a bar to prove which of them was the fittest.

'You'll be interested in this, Bernie', I was told. 'It's a bit of running, swimming and cycling.' It sounded fun. The only problem was that the event was in a month's time and the course was from London to Paris – running from London to Dover, swimming the Channel, and cycling from Calais to Paris, as you do. The race was fantastic. Although I hadn't had a chance to do any real preparation, I was with a good mate from the Marines, Mick

McCarthy, and we spurred and insulted each other on to the end. We also managed to pick up a trophy – for being the team that spent the longest swimming the Channel…

After reaching the finish line, I wanted to take part in more triathlons. So the next weekend I went in for a triathlon event in Reading, came sixth and once again found myself in a national team. This time, because it was a new sport to everybody in the world, I felt I had more of a chance than in the Nordic skiing, and eventually worked my way up to 25th in the world, and 12th in Europe.

Around this time I experienced one of the most difficult races of my life, in conditions that were testing for all the wrong reasons. A national newspaper, *The Times*, asked me to go to Nepal to challenge three local Gurkhas in the Annapurna Triathlon Challenge. This was going to be a tough ask in any case, racing against well-trained and climate-adapted local soldiers and things weren't helped when our arrival coincided with a violent uprising against King Birendra.

Our first three days were spent under curfew in the hotel during which time I somehow managed to get shot at.

Eventually things calmed down a bit and we were able to get on our flight to the event in Pokhara, at which point things got really scary – because at 20,000 feet we lost one of the engines of our twin-prop plane. And the mountain peaks on either side of the plane were a lot higher than 20,000 feet. I guess we shouldn't have been that surprised because we'd seen a guy banging away at the engine with a hammer just before we took off. And to cap it all, during the event itself I got dysentery. If ever there was a case of poor race preparation, this was it.

The demands of training for the triathlon were starting to get quite heavy, so the Marines – who seemed to have been quite pleased with the positive public profile I'd given them through my appearances on *Survival of the Fittest* – gave me four years off to concentrate on competing for the national triathlon team (my side of the bargain was that I helped the corps with a recruitment drive and was, if you like, a public face for the Marines).

During this time I was able to go over to the Commonwealth Games in Auckland, as triathlon captain – triathlon was making its first appearance, as a demonstration sport – and then in 1993 as the triathlon team manager. It was fantastic to be involved in such a young, still innocent, sport. And it felt like a justification for all the activities I'd really enjoyed since I was a kid. Back in the 1970s, when I took up jogging, I had been a freak. Now there was recognition for this mix of endurance sports – given the final seal of approval by its inclusion in the 2000 Sydney Olympics. I also got involved in an event which was called Conquer the Arctic, where you had to perform two tasks a day 350 miles inside the Arctic Circle.

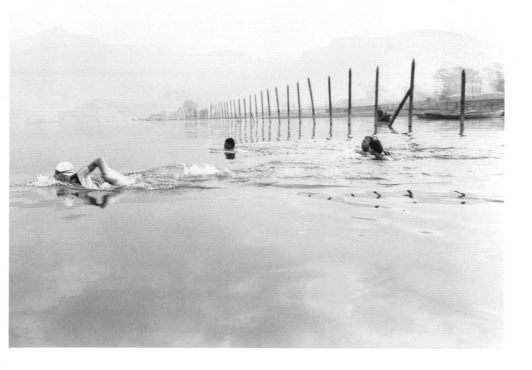

Still competing despite being shot at in Pokhara, Nepal

The Royal Marines taught me not to make excuses but just get on with it – that's what helped me later with my racing in the top end of sport.

This taught me more about teamwork. I was paired with a very, very good skier, but he couldn't work in the environment, sleeping out in snowholes; he simply wasn't used to operating as a team. He was just a normal bloke who wanted to get his head down in the warm after a difficult and exhausting day. What he didn't realise, since he had never had to do it before, was that you had to push yourself up another level, because with temperatures of –25°C outside, if we didn't dig that snowhole we wouldn't be competing the next day. Some of the other teams built ice caves, which meant the temperature was –10°C; I knew my snowhole would create a pretty toasty plus 5°C. But my colleague could not see that, and I really had to control myself

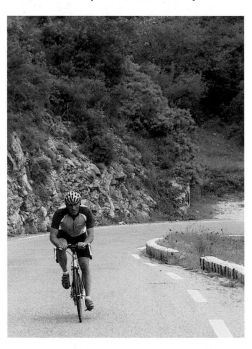

from not letting rip at him. I, only just, managed to remember that although I could have had a special forces guy with me who'd have gamely mucked in with digging that hole, he wouldn't have been that good at the physical techniques which we needed to complete the next day.

As my international competing days came to an end, I changed my life around. I'd got married in 1983 and wanted to concentrate on my family. I left the Marines and set up a personal fitness company in 1990 – corporate health, personal training, management training, interpersonal skills, that kind of thing. I enjoyed it, up to a point, but I was spending so much time on the business I hadn't realised how quickly my sharpness and fitness had disappeared, nor how much I missed regular sport and competition, until my wife Kim said in 1995, "You're getting uptight, Bernie – you need to be out there doing what you love most." She was right. Her comment got me back on track.

I started trying new activities, like rowing round Poole harbour in the early morning, and immediately found my appetite coming back.

In 1997 I had a call from the Prodrive Subaru World Rally team offering me the chance to take on a new challenge and direction by training world rally champion Colin McRae. From there (following Prodrive team boss Dave Richards) I moved to the Benetton Formula 1 team, which became the Renault F1 Team. I was now able to concentrate on becoming a 'human performance specialist' – a term that tries to get over what I think is

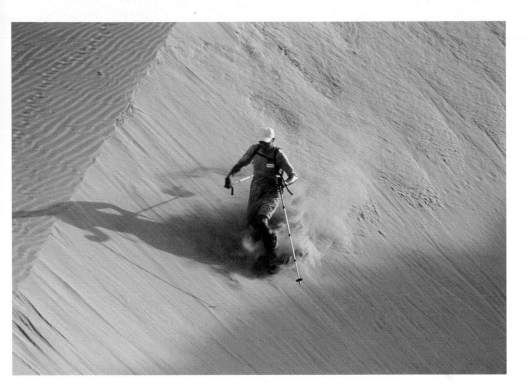

important in fitness, dealing with the body and the head, getting both to peak condition.

To me the word 'trainer' summons up a picture of a guy in a tracksuit with a bag and a sponge. What I hope you'll find in this book is that mental attitude and physical fitness are totally interlinked. My past experience also gave me the ideal opportunity to work with top-flight athletes, to try to pass on my enthusiasms and excitement, and of course to keep on learning.

Whether I'm involved in training for Formula 1, rallying or rowing, I always try to draw on my personal experiences and get inside the mind of the sportsmen and women I work with. Having been an international athlete I can understand the nerves, the fears, the pushing of limits: I'm able to get a long way inside the mind of any competitor. Which means that I can also cut the crap and get down to basics.

I like the story of Richard Burns, the rally driver: after an analysis of his psychological make-up and motivations and endless debates about what made a good driver great, he was told simply and directly by another driver, "You just need to drive faster, Richard."

Whether I'm talking to top-end sportspeople or club athletes, I always try to remember how an energetic young lad from Essex was able to improve himself by setting – and being given – achievable goals, so that the satisfaction of reaching each goal makes you want to carry on and reach the next one.

Everybody's personal targets are different, but the principles remain exactly the same, whether you just want to be slightly less out of breath in the Sunday League soccer match, or you want to complete a marathon. One of my personal goals is to compete in a coast-to-coast race in New Zealand, something I first

Jenson Button on an unusual endurance training session in Kenya

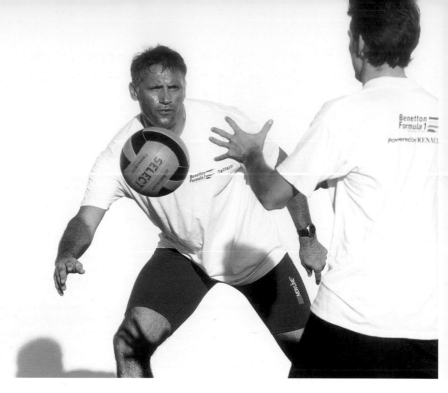

heard about when in Auckland at the Commonwealth Games in 1990. The event involves a mix of mountain running, trail running, cycling and white water paddling. I'm planning to do it before I'm 46, because I still relish the challenge and the environment.

And when I find a new challenge, as I have done recently by taking up canoeing again, I want to get really good at that sport, not just pelt up and down a river with no purpose. I want to tackle and master the rapids, sitting on a boiler (one of those parts of a rapid where the water is churning like crazy but not moving you anywhere), so that I can concentrate and look for the fastest line of attack.

However, I am not what I call a 'psycho trainer'. There are some trainers who like nothing better than to put you on a treadmill to hell, pushing your body so far that the experience is only about suffering. I've learnt that it's better to hit a zone where the feeling is one of intense pleasure, when the adrenalin kicks in,

and the euphoria takes over. That is not a sensation reserved for world-class athletes; you will be able to feel this too. You can feel that pleasure from a brisk walk in the park just as much as by completing a hill climb on a mountain bike. You are the yardstick to use, not other people's performance.

Being a member of a sports club or a fitness centre gives you many advantages: access to high quality equipment and advice and encouragement. But there is a downside. Looking at other people working out to extremes may make you feel as if you should be disappointed with your own performance; it all gets competitive and that only creates stress. Instead, remember that fitness is about pleasure not punishment, and about discovering your own capabilities.

I remember from my teens something important I learnt from doing the biathlon. Biathlon is a very demanding, actually very strange, discipline: a combination of some of the hardest cardiovascular

Jenson Button (back to camera) working with Bernie on his hand–eye coordination

When you start a training programme you may be disappointed about your early performance. Turn that disappointment into a plan for action.

exercise imaginable (the cross-country skiing) followed immediately by the need on the shooting range to achieve total body calm and mental discipline. What I learnt from participating in that sport was the ability to concentrate – and anyone who knows me knows that a gnat has a longer attention span.

First of all I had to understand that I needed to work on my weakness, i.e. my concentration, and then devise a strategy to deal with that and to help me block out any distractions. I spent a lot of time working on my focus, including exercises like standing on a chair on one leg (which definitely concentrates the mind) as well as controlled breathing exercises. Eventually I mastered the ability to swap from all-out exercise to total calm, and do it without falling over!

Colin McRae once told me that he also experienced this when he tried learning to fly a helicopter. He was so used to driving his rally car instinctively, with total control of the mechanical technique and without thinking about the process, that when he found himself in the helicopter cockpit where the controls were completely different, he had to force himself to develop the skill of concentration.

The other sport that I've been doing recently which has been giving me a lot of insight is K1 kayaking. A lot of beginners get stuck in and try to force the kayak round with brute strength and sheer muscle. What I have come to realise is that the sport is all about the combination of balance, technique, timing and – yet again – concentration, and that's what sorts the great from the good. I'm

certainly not great at kayaking, but I'm deriving a lot of pleasure from, once again, trying to analyse which areas of the sport I need to keep working on.

The reason I'm telling you all this is because one of the key messages I hope to get across in this book is that as well as mastering the mechanics of different exercises and workouts, I would like to encourage you to learn how to analyse what you need to achieve, where your weaknesses lie and how to counteract them. In other words, to ask yourself, 'Why am I doing this and where do I want to get to?' I'm not actually promising the path to enlightenment, but maybe we can find the sliproad...

With that in mind, that's enough about me and my story. Now let's concentrate on your fitness – we'll start by taking a look at how fit you are right now.

Now it's up to you.

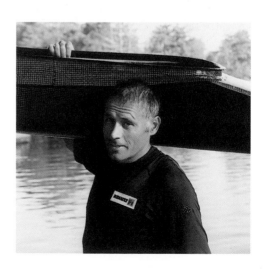

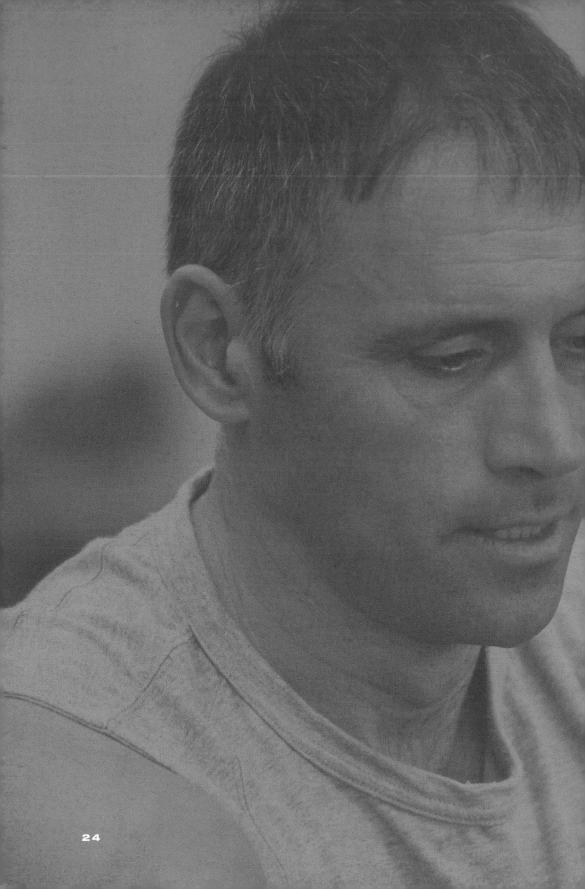

Shrosbree's six of the best
My favourite sports for getting fit

This section covers the main sports I have been heavily involved in over the last twenty-five years, both as a competitor and coach. They also happen to be my personal favourites. Without much formal academic training, I feel that I have come to understand the intricacies and subtleties of these sports, from technique to the psychological components, as well as all the training methods and principles involved. This has come from competing at international level in most of the sports and working with some of the the world's best athletes in each of the disciplines during my career.

I want to explain how I look at sport in a slightly different way to most people. At the moment my latest interest is K1 marathon paddling (see pages 62–67), an incredible sport which demands high levels of technique and fitness, and is practised in a beautiful environment. I love it because I am forced to think about the efficiency of my technique all the time and each session offers a challenge to keep progressing to another level. I often get out of the boat exhausted, not just because of the physical effort involved, but usually because of the mental effort I have had to put in to keep my balance and in reading the moving water. I find it difficult to concentrate on anything for more than a few minutes, but I can paddle intensely for 90 minutes, analysing virtually every paddle stroke in my head. Utterly immersed in what I'm doing.

I also want to get across the different types of conditioning that these sports have given me and how in many cases they have complemented each other. For instance, I know that reaching an international level standard in cross-country skiing and biathlon was an important factor in getting to the same level in triathlon. Cross-country skiing and biathlon gave me a solid base of endurance fitness but also the self-belief that having achieved international level in one sport, I could do it in another.

I'm far from unique in this approach: Alexander Popov used the principles of K1 paddling to enhance the fluidity of his freestyle swimming stroke and cyclist Greg Lemond often took to cross-country skiing trails over the winter to prepare for a summer of races which would include the Tour de France. What their attitude reveals is that you can look outside the traditional training you have always done for your sport and find other ways to enhance your performance and take it onto a new level.

The following sections on running, cycling, swimming, kayaking, rowing and cross-country skiing will give you the Bernie Shrosbree take on these sports, and, more importantly, show you how I try to get the most out of them and draw some inspiration from taking part. What you can do is apply my way of thinking to your own sport. Breaking the chain of traditional training often seems hard to accept – that is, until someone else has the courage to run with a new idea and create new standards in their particular sport.

Have you got it in you to break the training traditions in your sport?

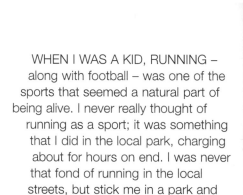

Running and walking

WHEN I WAS A KID, RUNNING – along with football – was one of the sports that seemed a natural part of being alive. I never really thought of running as a sport; it was something that I did in the local park, charging about for hours on end. I was never that fond of running in the local streets, but stick me in a park and I'd run till I dropped.

Later on I was inspired by the great British runners of the 1970s: legends like Dave Bedford, Brendan Foster and Ian Thompson. Their success – and later that of Coe, Ovett and Cram – was an essential part of the great boom in running awareness in the UK in the 70s and 80s. Everybody seemed to be into it.

But in the early 70s, when I started to go running seriously near my home, wearing shorts and a vest, I can remember people shouting 'Weirdo', and 'What's the matter with you, mate?' For some reason they seemed to think that running was an alien activity if it took place outside school or the Olympics. But since Run the World in the mid-80s, the rise of mini, half and full marathons has given a credibility, a structure and a network of support for anyone who wants to run – at any level.

Running has played a major role in my life: cross-country events at school, joining the local athletics club, fell running in Scotland with a bunch of Marines, taking part in triathlon. In the 1990s one of

Winning a New Year's day 10k race

In the early 70s, when I started to go running seriously near my home, I can remember people shouting 'Weirdo'. Well, we're all weirdos now.

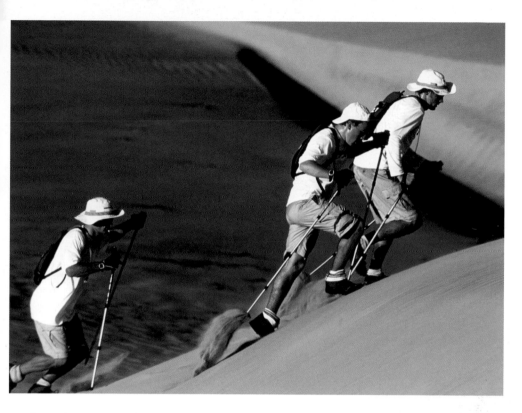

my favourite runs was from Lulworth Cove to Osmington and back, followed by a dive in the sea (even in winter) and a big old breakfast at the local cafe.

There are all sorts of ways to run and it is also a simple and relatively cheap sport in which to participate – after all, the environment comes free of charge so make the most of it. I always carry a running kit in the back of the car and if I've had a meeting somewhere I drive to a suitable place, stop in a car park, change – Superman-style – into my running kit and head off into a park or some hills for an hour or two.

Running and walking include five distinct areas:

1 Jogging
2 Endurance running
3 Race-specific or competitive running
4 Sprinting
5 Walking

JOGGING

Is at the light intensity end of running and is all about gently working the heart and lungs. When you are jogging you should be able to hold a conversation with your running partner and, at the end of the jog, your legs should feel heavy – but not wiped out.

Remember, each time your foot lands

Trulli, Alonso and Button work hard at sand dune training in Kenya

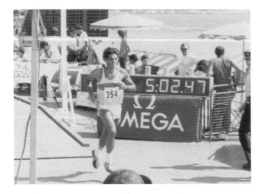

back on the ground, so does the rest of your weight, which is why jogging can turn out to be a big disappointment for some people. As your weight comes down on the load-bearing joints, they have to take the strain, and if you begin running at too high an intensity, too quickly, you can find yourself spending a lot of time at the physio's.

The jogging boom of the 70s and 80s has dwindled a little, but the interest remains. Jogging is easy, it's convenient and rewarding in terms of the considerable fitness gains you can make. Think of jogging as a conditioning phase for other forms of running, and keep the intensity low. Start slowly and don't kill yourself. If you have set yourself a regular distance to run and it's proving painful, it is much more valuable to run halfway and walk the rest of the way, or jog for two minutes and walk for one, rather than pushing yourself to exhaustion and never going out again.

If you're jogging in a hilly area and you come across a steep incline, drop back to brisk walking until the ground levels out again.

Keep reviewing your performances and

think about which part of your body is aching next morning, and it will ache – you're pounding three to four times your body weight through your poor old kneecaps. And then add some complementary weight training at the gym. Step-ups (see page 192), or even joining a step class, will help a lot. Or use the indoor cycle to strengthen your quads and hamstrings.

Jogging is routinely used to complement other sports either before serious training starts or as an active recovery or cool down option.

Brisk walks or light jogs are great for mobility and the best example I saw of this was at Bath Rugby Club. On Monday mornings, after the weekend match, the players would struggle out of the changing room – assuming they weren't lying on the physio's slab – and onto the training pitch as if they were coming back from a war zone. After a walk and jog and some mobility work, they would get stuck right back into intensive drills and skill sessions.

Over the years I've put my body through a lot and as I've got older and long since moved out of the spring chicken category, I find I suffer from a range of aches and pains the day after a hard training session. But a recovery jog or brisk walk soon shakes them off and what better way to start the day than gently cantering through the open fields?

Neil Bowman, my cross-country ski coach, would have us up at six o'clock in the morning in the middle of winter in Norway, wrapped up like Eskimos and out the lodge to walk and jog in temperatures of –20°C or worse, to help wake up the body before an eight-thirty start for either a biathlon or cross-country ski race.

I still use this approach with drivers today. Carlos Sainz, the World Rally champion, would not always perform at his best on the early morning stages of the WRC (the stages used to sometimes begin at five-thirty), but once we set up a routine of either a 15-minute swim or a short jog before he climbed into the cockpit, his performances during those crucial early morning stages improved dramatically.

ENDURANCE RUNNING

I think of this type of running as part of the basic conditioning phase for all sorts of different sports, particularly those such as football and rugby where running and spending a lot of time on your feet are an inevitable part of the game. Those of you who take part in other non-weight-bearing sports can gain a lot from some running conditioning too; it gets swimmers away from the monotony of staring at the black line at the bottom of the pool and is one of the best activities to help control body weight in sports such as martial arts or boxing.

Regular conditioning runs are a stage on from jogging and are generally performed at about Level 3 on the Shrosbree Perceived Exertion Scale (see page 241), i.e. you know you are working, but it still feels pretty comfortable. The considerable fitness gains that accrue from endurance running come from the amount of time you spend on the road or trail and in the regularity of the sessions, and emphatically not from how high an intensity you work.

Arthur Lydiard, the great New Zealand coach who produced some of the best distance runners of the 60s and 70s, had a simple but hugely successful philosophy of 'just get the miles in', which will still work very well today.

Most running injuries occur because of training too hard and can be avoided by sticking to sensible levels of activity. If you're using running as basic conditioning for other non-running sports, there is little reason to be doing interval sessions and sprint workouts (unless you're a very serious footballer, rugby player, or play competitive racquet sports). These are great training sessions to tease top performance out of your body, but they can also put you on the knife edge of injury or illness. Ask yourself if it is really worth the risk when you can improve your fitness considerably by concentrating on plenty of steady-paced training.

For my own conditioning running – when I'm not training specifically for a race or event – I much prefer to get out on the trails and up in the hills rather than pounding the streets. This gives me a better all-round condition as it strengthens ankles and knees on the uneven ground and above all it gets me out into the environment I love most. Put it this way, if you're out there running at a comfortable pace, taking in the scenery and coming home feeling elated and nicely weary, that is what conditioning running is all about.

Endurance running has been a vital part of my life, my fitness as well as the most enjoyable of all the sports I've been involved in. I don't envy those of you that have to fit your training in before and after work or

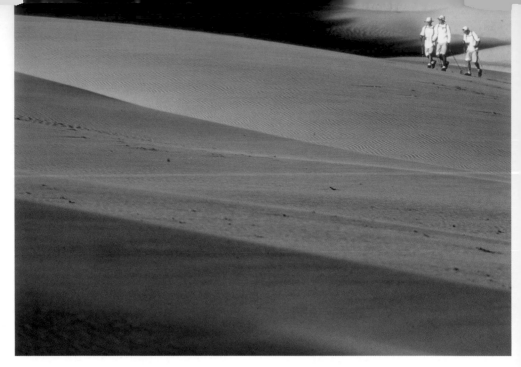

anyone who has to train in an urban environment – perhaps preparing for a marathon or local race. But I hope that you treat yourself when you can and get out onto the hills and mountains, the trails and the coastal paths. The tranquillity of endurance running is second to none and the sheer joy of venturing out onto remote trails where it's just you, the environment and the elements, whether for forty minutes or four hours, will give you massive motivational as well as conditioning benefits.

RACE-SPECIFIC OR COMPETITIVE RUNNING

This is where running becomes a sport in its own right. The diversity of distances and types of terrain mean that there really is something for everyone out there and I reckon in my career I've had a go at most of them! The basic conditioning running described in the last section forms the basis of training for all of the following disciplines with some specific variations to fine tune your fitness for your chosen event.

The track is the most focused and competitive form of running and takes place over distances from 800m to 10,000m (anything less than 800m is considered a sprint). If you are wanting to get into track racing the only way is to join a decent athletics club. There's bound to be one in your area and they will be able to point you in the right direction. The training required to be competitive on the track revolves around large amounts of conditioning-type running with speed intervals, technique drills and sprint work to get the body ready for these fast and furious types of races. There are few people who train on the track purely for fitness – it's more a place for competitive athletes – so unless that's what you're after it might be best to look at some of the more relaxed types of running below.

My own experience of track racing came when, as part of my cross-country ski summer training, I raced the 1500m for the Marines in the Interservices Championships against some of Britain's top runners of the time, including Steve Jones and Chris Robinson. Even as a top skier, racing against these elite runners was an intimidating prospect, and one that would prove (or disprove) whether my fitness gained from my own sport would transfer to another. With a few specific track training sessions to build the leg speed and lactate tolerance I needed for an event lasting less than four minutes, I was able to step up and race with these guys. Even if I was not in a position to beat them I could, nonetheless, compete and get in amongst the race.

It also taught me a great lesson in mental toughness. I was probably better suited to the 5,000m or 10,000m after all the long endurance skiing I'd done, but I knew that subjecting myself to the shorter distance and faster paced race would really test me mentally and physically by forcing me into a deep, dark hole of pain. I was more nervous standing on the start line than at the World Championships because I knew what I was going to have to do to myself to hang on for a respectable time.

and train, as the sessions are set and you feel like you have to be there. It also adds to the enjoyment factor for a lot of people; we've all heard about the loneliness of the long-distance runner…

Joining a local club is probably also the best way to progress from jogging or conditioning-type running to participating or racing in organised events. You'll get information about local events and feel the camaraderie of running with your team, which all adds to the overall experience.

Sometimes, and I've often seen it with club runners, there can be a downside to group training and club sessions. They can turn into mini-races or ego-flexing sessions, where some guys like to really push the pace on (and surprisingly enough it is often the men who are most guilty of this). What then happens is that you end up making the grave mistake of training for the session and not the goal you are aiming for; you end up running too hard and burning out before race day.

Road running is by far the most popular form of running generally. There are races every weekend, and some midweek, from marathons right down to 5km (3 mile) fun runs.

A lot of people like to join clubs to do group training sessions and go to races with clubmates, making it a social part of life. Group training can be great for people who lack a little bit of self-motivation to get out

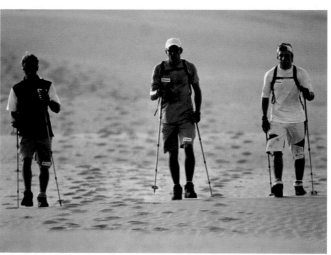

Hiking: the poles help speed and strengthen the shoulders and back

There's a time and a place for pushing yourself in training, but don't get involved in this type of competition-driven punishment all of the time. It will only end in tears.

The final word on road running must be one of caution. Too many runners get silly, niggling injuries by training too hard and putting in too many miles on the road. Shin splints (painful and tender shins) and soreness in muscles and joints are very common as people pile on the miles, training for marathons and other long races. Some sensible off-road training, alternative sessions like swimming and cycling combined with moderate road running, will keep you out there training more consistently and give you much better all-round fitness than filling the diary with huge amounts of tarmac-flattening miles. I ran some of my best road running times (which were national class at the time) off the back of only three to four quite intensive running sessions a week, as I was also swimming and cycling for triathlon at the time.

Just thought I'd drop that in to get you high-mileage junkies thinking...

Off-road running: nowadays I do almost all of my running off-road. I would describe fell running, trail running and cross-country running as some of the finest forms of training there are (in the same way the great coach Arthur Lydiard considered off-road running a key part of the training for all his athletes). You get all the aerobic benefits of running while having to concentrate on the terrain all of the time, dancing over loose rocks and being out in the natural environment. You build up strength in the joints, stabilise the muscles in your trunk and get more variety in the gradients to spice up your sessions.

However, the type of fitness you get from this training is very specific. Joss Naylor, one of the great fell runners, was reasonably good on the road but not spectacular. The reverse is often true and elite track runners don't always transfer their talent successfully into the country because their sense of balance and specific muscle strength is geared to motoring round a flat surface rather than an uneven one. That's why, if you are serious about your running, a healthy mix of disciplines is good, but you need to focus most of your training on the terrain you are going to be competing on.

There are some great off-road events which take place mainly over the winter season, from cross-countries that are generally on pretty tame courses (fields and tracks) right through to extreme fell races that require river crossings and semi-scrambling-type climbs and descents to test your nerves as much as your fitness. Again a local club is your

Bernie's tip
If you enjoy walking to the point that you are seriously considering taking up race walking, then make sure you join a club and get expert tuition. Race walking is a very technical and demanding sport, so you need a high level of coaching.

best bet for finding these events and the emphasis is as much on taking part and completing the course as it is on racing.

I have some great memories of the extreme fell running we did in *Survival of the Fittest* where we raced up and down some huge mountains in the UK and North America. There was this crazy American 'dude' who in the interview before the downhill scree run was stating how he'd 'do anything to win' including 'risk life and limb to make sure I'm first over the line'.

True to his word, the guy literally threw himself down the run like a rag doll and fell over the line, smashing up his hip and requiring stitches in his face and hands. Of course, the minor problem with his approach was that it put him out of the rest of the competition! I think he's now a hero to the *Jackass* generation.

Distance running technique

As running is a pretty natural movement for most of us, you might not have considered that there is a lot of technique involved. It's true that generally most runners move in an instinctive way and altering that too much may go against inbuilt mechanics. But there are some basic parts of the running 'gait' that can be looked at to enhance performance. These are:

- Stride length
- Turnover
- Knee lift

Stride length will depend a lot on your leg length and flexibility. Despite what you might think, longer strides are not necessarily better, although shuffling along with little fairy steps probably won't get you round the London Marathon alongside Paula Radcliffe. To find optimum stride length, I used to go down to the beach and do some timed runs so that I could see the stride patterns I made in soft sand. I'd experiment with different patterns to see if altering the length of each step made me feel and move more efficiently. This is hardly the most scientific assessment, I know – and these days you could probably get it done in the sports lab – but it got me thinking about and feeling the differences stride length could make, and helped me get close to my own optimum. It's worth a try if you're getting into your running a bit more seriously and want to get the best out of your performance.

Turnover refers to the cadence of your legs. Some people call it 'leg speed'. It is an important performance factor in racing, where your ability to run economically and smoothly at a fast pace is crucial. To highlight what I mean, imagine the guy who does loads of hard training runs on heavy, hilly cross-country courses and gets incredibly strong and fit, but never actually runs at a fast pace. Stick him in a fast road run and he'll get crucified, because at the neuromuscular level (the brain-to-muscle connections) his legs aren't used to the quick turnover required and they fatigue much sooner than the rest of his system.

A great way to train for turnover is downhill running on a subtle, smooth gradient or on the flat with wind assistance. Sessions for turnover don't have to be

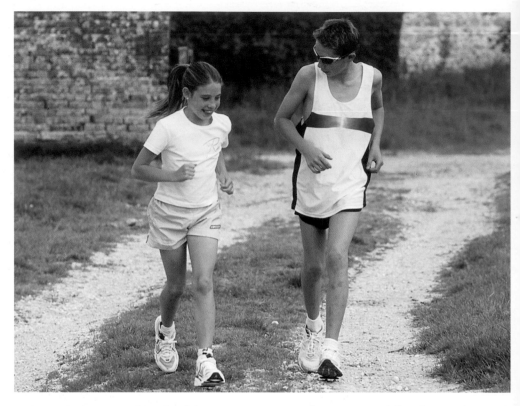

arduous, but you need to stimulate your muscles to fire up at a rate that equates to a bit above race pace, which grows the nerve pathways to the muscles so that your legs 'learn' to run quickly.

Knee lift: I have always used high knee drills in sand dunes and on steep hills to increase strength in the hip area and improve the toe-off aspect of my running. Back down at the beach, running in shallow water is another great way to enhance your knee lift: if you don't lift your knees high enough you end up tripping over yourself and going for an unscheduled swim. If you find yourself

struggling on steep hills when racing, these kinds of drills might help increase your specific strength in this area of your performance.

Finally, a word on breathing technique for running. I was first asked about it when I ran coaching courses for triathletes; until then I had honestly never really thought about it. Running is all about relaxation in your body from the waist up, and if you're concentrating too hard on breathing the chances are you will just tense up. When you're working really hard on a steep incline, you might find it helpful to exhale forcefully in time with your steps to stabilise your core and power up the climb, but this is really the only time you should be concerned with what your lungs are doing. Try to keep relaxed and focused on rhythm as the main priority.

SPRINTING

60m, 100m, 200m and 400m are the classic sprint events in athletics. They require a different approach to training when compared with distance running as the way energy is supplied to the muscles is totally different. Power, technique and range of movement are the most important factors in sprint training, so lifting weights, doing technique drills and stretching form a huge part of a sprinter's programme.

To reach a high level in sprinting requires a certain body type (tall and muscular) with a large percentage of 'fast twitch muscle fibres'. These fibres are able to produce high levels of force quickly, but they also tire quickly. Slow twitch muscle fibres on the other hand produce less force but keep going for longer, making them better suited to distance events. Although training can shift the balance of slow and fast twitch muscle fibres slightly, your genetic start point will determine how far you can go and explains the comment by an eminent sports physiologist that 'If you want to be an Olympic gold medallist you had better choose your parents very carefully!'

As sprinting is so highly technical, good coaching is essential. An expert second pair of eyes is vital for evaluating form and technique so that all the power being applied to the track maximises forward motion.

The role of sprint training in diverse sports such as rugby and bobsleigh has become more prominent in recent years, as we've seen ex-sprinters coming across from athletics to compete and coach in these events. I did some work with Bath Rugby Club when England player Mike Tindall was coming back from a knee injury. After his basic physiotherapy rehab was well under way, we did some weightlifting and explosive sprint drills to start bringing his speed and agility back. We did some straight-line running as well as timed gated runs; when we had finished it looked like a racehorse had been churning up the grass because of the power Mike was putting into each turn to decelerate and accelerate back up to speed again!

Like other forms of track running, sprinting is best done at an organised athletics club, so if you fancy yourself as the next Linford Christie (and I'm not talking about the size of your lunchbox) get down to your local track to take some proper advice.

WALKING

Fifteen years ago, when I was competing regularly, if somebody had said to me that walking was a way to get fit, I'd have turned my nose up at it; I had a very blinkered view at the time of what fitness training involved. Now I have come to realise that walking plays a fundamental role in conditioning training. Not least, it's a great starting point for building up your confidence, if you've been out of the fitness loop for a while or you were never that keen on sports, because it allows you to start achieving small, short-time goals including weight loss.

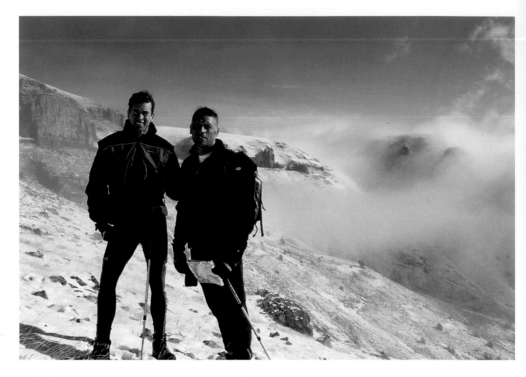

A simple example: my father, who had been a talented cyclist, lost the fitness habit by the time he was in his late 30s. He had a family and was on shift work at Ford's in Dagenham. All the fitness he'd had when he was younger – and had probably taken for granted – started to fall away, and his eating habits were not that good in terms of nutritional value. He was getting unhealthy and feeling it. Some friends asked him to play football, but after ten years without any real exercise, and a few extra pounds around his middle, he felt embarrassed and made excuses to get out of it. Off his own back he decided to do something about his fitness level and to change his lifestyle. He began walking to work as well as walking

regularly round one of the nearby parks. Gradually he was able to see an improvement, so much so that he went on to complete three marathons.

Walking is a great stepping-stone towards future fitness. Don't underestimate its value. If you can manage three or four brisk walks a week, with a two-hour walk at the weekend, you will notice a major improvement in your fitness after just six weeks or so. You can also take it at your own pace initially without any likelihood of seriously injuring yourself, and then start to increase the difficulty factor as you want, either walking for longer, or faster, up steeper gradients or carrying weights. The benefits of walking include:

– improving your cardiovascular efficiency
– helping prevent osteoporosis (brittle bones) in later life
– improving your all-round mobility
– perfect for the older age ranges or for returning to fitness after a layoff

And you don't have to go to the Peak or Lake Districts to do it (although both of those areas are fabulous places to enjoy walking). Most parks have some kind of trail. Or if you're a golfer, you can make sure you're walking briskly up gradients and getting extra exercise during a round.

I personally love to walk along the coastal paths in Dorset. Ramblers have long appreciated the benefits of walking and taking in the ambience of the countryside. The first time you tackle a ramble with heavy boots and a backpack, you usually can't wait until the end of the day to relax, soak your feet and have a beer. After a few walks, however, you'll notice that the aches in your back, hips and neck are less noticeable, as the Longer, Lower, Regular (see page 98) nature of country walking starts working on your body.

In the gym, the treadmill is a standard piece of equipment, but like so many bits of kit, most people have no idea how to use it: you can see people pounding away at a rate of knots looking like they're on the Great March and apparently close to exhaustion.

Always start at a sensible intensity – 5km an hour is good for most people – and then gradually, gradually build that up to a brisk walk, before increasing the gradient (again, gradually) so that more muscle groups come into play, including your back and shoulders (see pages 100–103).

Equipment: most joggers underdress or overdress. At one end of the spectrum is the plastic bag club, who wear ten waterproof jackets and an array of hats. This is the old boxing mentality – sweat it all out. But although you can see some short-term weight loss (which is precisely the reason why boxers used to rely on it, of course), dehydration is a much more likely side-effect, and a high level of fluid loss can lead to headaches and kidney infections. However, if you underdress, swanning around the park in midwinter in a flimsy top and shorts, you'll just catch a chill.

In autumn and winter I recommend wearing a long pair of lightweight running tights, a long-sleeved thermal top, with a windproof vest, lightweight jacket or sweatshirt over that. A hat and headband in the cold and the wind will stop you catching a head cold. Gloves will also stop your extremities getting cold. In spring and summer, thigh-length running shorts with a T-shirt or running vest is fine, although it is always better to overdress and then take off one layer – scrunch up a lightweight jacket or tie it round your waist – than to run the risk of being chilled, as cold muscles are susceptible to injury.

As far as running shoes go, I always suggest that you go to a specialist running store, rather than a high street sports outfitter, where they will most likely sell you the pair of shoes with the highest mark-up: you'd be better off running in slippers. Go for a heavy to mid-weight shoe that will absorb all the shocks of running. They might not look quite so fashionable but they will save your hips and your knees.

Progression in your training

The 10km running chart

WHERE A LOT OF COMPETITIVE athletes – in all sports, not just running – can fall down is in the progression of their training, or more accurately the lack of it. All of us would like to improve our personal bests or move up a few places in our age group, but this is actually quite hard to do. Which is why, when you look over the results of local races from the last few years, many decent club athletes will be knocking out roughly the same times year after year, making little improvement.

Is this because most people are at their peak already and have no room for improvements? Probably not. More likely the same old approach to training is being employed and the same old results are, therefore, inevitable.

It's the same for those who design their training too precisely. According to their immaculate training plan, these athletes reckon that they will know what their heart rate will be in the twenty-seventh minute of their run in six weeks' time. They put together a scientifically sound programme that sadly fails to include the flexibility to deal with their almost inevitable failure to meet all the programme's targets – which is what happens in the real world. Usually this leads to the programme hitting the bin and training resuming as per usual. While a planned approach is definitely required to get to where you want to be, the real skill lies in being able to constantly review the short-term, session-by-session goals

while still keeping the big picture in focus.

Why is achieving progression so hard? Because it's often not a linear process. You might start training from scratch and the improvements in your performance will be impressive, all without too much thought – just doing something physical will have a dramatic effect on an untrained body. Sooner or later, though, you will need to change your training as your body adapts to it. When a plateau like this occurs it can really knock your motivation if you don't know how to tweak up the pressure to get the body to adapt further.

Sometimes you might find your fitness drops away because of illness, injury, loss of motivation or even overtraining. Coming back from a loss of physical form like this needs careful management; you should build up slowly and not expect to get back to your highest heights in a week if you've been laid up for ten days with the 'flu.

At international level the margins are much tighter. Improvements might be limited to one or two percent, but this can represent the difference between being a medallist or an also ran. At this level it can take years to make headway – look at how many seasons Paula Radcliffe spent getting into the top five, but never actually winning. Many factors go into great achievements such as hers, but a steady, patient process of progression is what it is all based on. You will experience ups and downs in performance, but what you want

Looking for 1 second a week over a kilometre doesn't sound like much, but it allows the body to adapt slowly and progressively.

to see over a significant period of time is progression which is not always evident from week to week, even month to month, but over the long term gets you to where you want to be.

The running times chart (on page 41) was devised by Paul Hart, a runner who has coached some fantastic athletes from the 70s onwards. Paul is from the great era of British distance running and has a wealth of experience which was used to generate this chart. It wasn't cooked up in some sports science lab: all the times here have been run over and over again by a lot of athletes and it has helped all levels of runners achieve their goals.

This chart was initially based on the performances of three main athletes. First was Roger Matthews, who was British 10,000 metres champion and ran to 4th place in the 1970 Commonwealth Games The top level (Level 18) was tried and tested by Roger and Paul in 1970. Second was Brent Jones, a runner who trained under Paul from the age of 15 to 23, when a chronic back injury forced his untimely retirement. Brent started in at about Level 13 and progressed to Level 17 over the years. And Paul himself has tried and tested levels from Level 13 to Level 16, and more recently reckons he's moved steadily back down to Level 1! What this shows is that the times and training sessions that have generated the chart have a history and substance, founded on experience – rather than pure theory.

The basic idea is to progress through the levels of the interval training (or similar sessions) at the set pace/times indicated,

reducing the recovery between each repetition (rep) over the weeks. When you progress to the next level you return to the full recovery time, reducing it bit by bit over the next few week and so on. As you can see, the improvements are only about 5 seconds per kilometre and with the time that this takes to move up a level (4–6 weeks) you are only looking for 1 second a week over a kilometre! That doesn't sound like much, but it allows the body to adapt slowly and progressively, reducing injury and overtraining risks, as well as ensuring a good long-term progression. Sounds great doesn't it, but it's not always that simple. The key is managing the progression of the training as it won't ever be as simple or as direct as a 1 second a week improvement. Fluctuations in mood, form, fitness, diet and weather can play havoc with that. However, if you get the 5 seconds over 4–6 weeks or 10 seconds over 2 months, you will have made real progress, even if from time to time the weekly sessions are up and down a bit. The exact sessions like 5 x 1000m, for instance, are not set in stone by any means. Mixing them up and varying the distances run by doing 6 x 800m or 3 x 1600m, for example, can provide a bit of variety and increase the range of your abilities, or you can increase the pace slightly to change the stress on the body and mind to keep it interesting. Also, substituting efforts such as 5 x 3min instead of 5 x 1000m once in a while will give you a great training effect without the self-induced pressure of hitting your target times week in, week out. It should also go without saying that these sessions are

> **Bernie's tip**
> Reading this once, you might find it a bit complicated. But stick with it. For those of you trying to find the gain in competitive performance it will deliver, I promise.

only one part of your weekly training routine complementing long runs, steady state efforts, as well as any other training you might be doing.

The chart is designed to help you to move forward in a progressive way. It's not an exact blueprint, nor does it guarantee success, and it is not a pattern to follow religiously week in week out.

What you can do, though, is to drop in elements of the kind of training it is based on and use it at key times of the year to build up to a peak for your big events. If you are not a runner, the chart should still be of use since the ideas it represents are applicable to other events and the concept is valid across all sorts of sports. You just have to think about how you want to apply the idea to your sport.

To explain the chart, working from left to right:
– the Level number is a reference for each stage and covers speeds from jogging up to international running.
– the 10km time is your current level of performance from a recent race or time trial.
– Pace/K represents what your 10km race time equates to in minutes per kilometre.
– the eq 5km time gives an approximation of the time you can reasonably expect to run 5km in a race based on your 10km time. This is obviously slightly quicker than half of the 10km time. Again the pace/K equates to your 5km pace per kilometre.
– next comes the approximation of your 3km race pace ability, slightly quicker than 5km pace.
– the next three columns are indicators of

what pace your training sessions of 5 x 1000m, 2 x 2000m and 3 x 3000m should (roughly) be performed at, with appropriate recovery times listed at the bottom of each column. Reducing the recovery time is one way of increasing the overload of the sessions, as is increasing the pace of the rep, but beware of trying to do both at once (i.e. running quicker with less recovery time): this leads to disappointment and massive overload with injury and illness round the corner.

I would also encourage you to play around with the different surfaces and terrains you run on and the format of the sessions. If you vary these elements of your sessions fairly regularly you won't find them becoming so monotonous and end up unnecessarily competing against yourself and the session. If you can avoid always lapping the same old track, a few seconds here and there becomes a lot less significant and will make your training a lot less stressful.

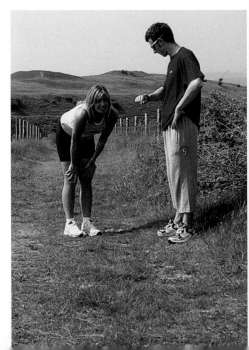

10k stepping stones

Level	10K time	Pace/K	eq 5K time	Pace/K	eq 3K	5x1000	4x2000	3x3000
L1	45:00	4:30	21:40	4:20	12:20	@ 4:07	@ 8:50	@ 13:30
L2	44:00	4:24	20:50	4:10	12:00	@ 4:00	@ 8:35	@ 13:12
L3	43:00	4:18	20:20	4:04	11:45	@ 3:55	@ 8:22	@ 12:54
L4	42:00	4:12	19:55	3:59	11:30	@ 3:50	@ 8:12	@ 12:36
L5	41:00	4:06	19:30	3:55	11:15	@ 3:45	@ 8:02	@ 12:18
L6	40:00	4:00	19:00	3:48	11:00	@ 3:40	@ 7:48	@ 12:00
L7	39:00	3:54	18:30	3:42	10:30	@ 3:30	@ 7:36	@ 11:42
L8	38:00	3:48	18:00	3:36	10:15	@ 3:25	@ 7:24	@ 11:24
L9	37:00	3:42	17:30	3:30	10:00	@ 3:20	@ 7:12	@ 11:06
L10	36:00	3:36	17:00	3:24	9:45	@ 3:15	@ 7:00	@ 10:48
L11	35:00	3:30	16:30	3:18	9:30	@ 3:10	@ 6:48	@ 10:30
L12	34:00	3:24	16:00	3:12	9:15	@ 3:03	@ 6:36	@ 10:12
L13	33:00	3:18	15:40	3:08	9:03	@ 3:01	@ 6:26	@ 9:54
L14	32:00	3:12	15:10	3:02	8:45	@ 2:55	@ 6:14	@ 9:36
L15	31:00	3:06	14:45	2:57	8:30	@ 2:50	@ 6:04	@ 9:18
L16	30:00	3:00	14:15	2:51	8:15	@ 2:45	@ 5:50	@ 9:00
L17	29:00	2:54	13:45	2:45	8:00	@ 2:40	@ 5:40	@ 8:42
L18	28:00	2:48	13:15	2:39	7:45	@ 2:35	@ 5:30	@ 8:24
						4 down to 1 min recovery	5 down to 2 min recovery	5 min recovery

Cycling

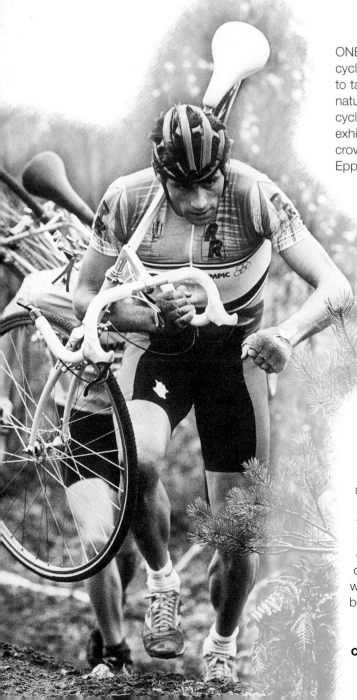

ONE OF THE GREAT THINGS ABOUT cycling is that it is a fantastic opportunity to take yourself and your bike out into the natural environment. When I first started cycling seriously, I found it completely exhilarating to be able to get away from crowded streets into the clean air of Epping Forest.

Cycling was something of a family tradition for the Shrosbrees: my father and mother were both keen, club standard riders. So it was relatively natural for me to want to take up the sport, although I think I would have done so anyway: I seem to have a natural affinity with bikes. And in terms of fitness, there are so many benefits.

Cycling is a very safe way to build up your basic conditioning, especially if you're coming back into training and exercise after losing the habit for a while – or after an injury has sidelined you from your usual sport.

It is also not weight bearing, and that is particularly important if you're older or on the heavy side: it's much easier on the joints. That means you can exercise for longer, work on any weight loss you want to achieve, and boost your cardiovascular efficiency.

Cyclo-cross racing near the New Forest in

And once you've got your cycling technique working smoothly you should be able to carry on cycling till ... well, I've got friends who are cycling regularly well into their 80s, still supple and still energetic.

Cycling is a sport for life. And you can share the fun of it with your family and friends. I love hooking up with a bunch of guys I raced with ten years or so ago. We'll meet up, have a good workout with a 50-mile ride together and then treat ourselves to a mug of tea or, if it's hot, a swift half in a country pub to finish.

Apart from the social side, cycling is one of those sports that allows you plenty of time to think as you're doing it. You can concentrate on your technique – the 'ankling' or 'souplesse' – and try to improve that while you're pedalling.

Or you can simply enjoy the pleasure of working with your bike. You are the one who's providing all the power to climb a mountain in the Alps for two and a half hours: your reward is descending the same hill at speed in a fifth of the time.

When you and your bike are working perfectly, you can hear the machinery singing along. It's a natural high; your body starts releasing endorphins. You don't have to be a world-class athlete to achieve this. You'll just feel like one!

And if you want to increase the exhilaration factor then go mountain biking. I have always loved the smell of pine forests and the rocks – especially granite: a marvellous smell I first discovered on an archaeology trip when I was at school. It makes the high street seem pretty grim.

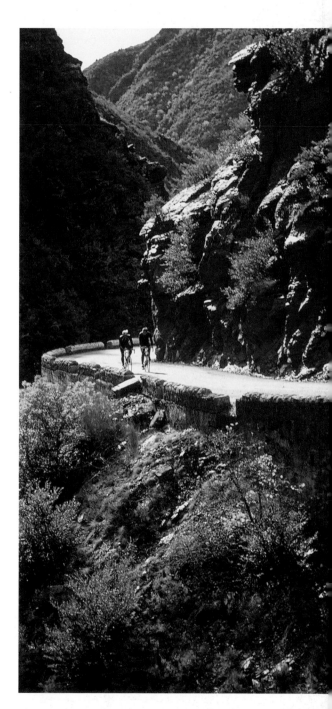

Riding with Ralph Firman in the Maritime Alps

I started mountain biking in the mid 80s when the bikes first started arriving in the United Kingdom and I still enjoy the sport today. Frankly, there are few sports more exhilarating now that the technology of the bikes has really come on. It is hugely enjoyable to power through moorland or descend hilly terrain at breathtaking speed. Then there are long demanding climbs that have a real psychological aspect to them. Will you cope? How far can you get up this great big hill without getting off the bike – using your skills, the bike's technology and your own physical effort? Mountain bike racing is now a very serious sport in which speed, technical ability, endurance and perfect balance on the bike are all tested. I enjoy coaching people in this field, but if you just want to get out there on forest trails, and get around the countryside better than riding around the lanes, nothing can beat mountain biking. It's one sport I don't care what the weather is like, I'll go out in sleet, snow, hail, wind and rain – it's great!

Some people don't like cycling. And there's no reason why you should. Other people have a dislike for running, rowing or swimming. Usually I find this is because they have not been conditioned for that sport, and their initial exposure to it has been difficult, negative and even painful. That applies equally to cycling.

Cycling has suffered from being seen for a long time as a second-class means of transport, just something holding up the traffic – and although cycle paths and lanes are becoming more common, the cycling experience on the road is often far from comfortable or healthy.

I also think that we have often learnt to ride a bike badly. There's rarely any teaching, just your dad running alongside you when you're a kid before launching you off, hopefully, into the distance. The expression that does all the damage is that one about something being 'as easy as riding a bike'. Actually, to ride a bike well is both difficult and hard work.

When I first took up the triathlon in 1984, it took me 27 minutes to complete a 10-mile time trial. I thought I was fit – in

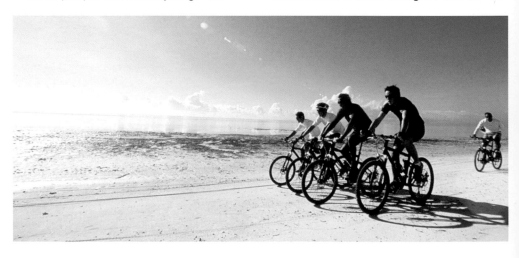

44   **The Renault F1 Team cruise into the pit lane, Kenya**

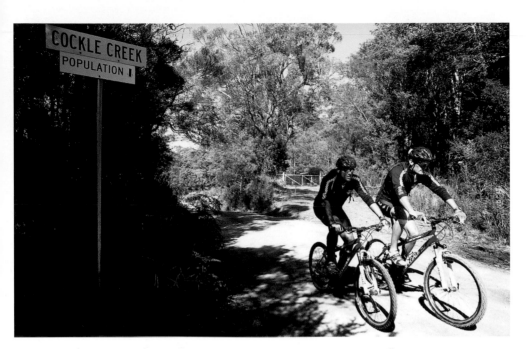

fact I thought I was very fit – but even so, I couldn't move after I finished the trial, because I was so stiff. Eventually I was able to improve my time by developing an understanding of the mechanism of the bike and the psychological side of cycling.

That understanding doesn't have to be scientific; it can be completely instinctive. I was cycling once with some good mates, including Mark Fodden, a builder who has real grit. We were out on a bike ride one evening on a 70-mile run, and at one point on the valley road heading towards Dorchester, we'd adopted an aerodynamic 'echelon' formation. I was the only one with a computer on the bike. After about eight miles I looked down and the computer told me we were doing 33mph. Mark dropped off behind me for about fifteen seconds and said, "Step on the gas, Bernie." I looked down and the reading was 32mph! Mark had sensed that slight drop in speed without having to resort to any technology.

If you're going to take up road racing you need that sense of pace – if you drift even a couple of feet off the pace you can lose it big time. So you are constantly monitoring your pace and how it compares with the efforts of the other riders; another example of the constant mind games that you have to play, which stop you ever getting bored in the saddle.

The cross-training potential of cycling is exceptional. When I began working with former World Champion Rally driver Colin McRae he had not done much, if any, cycling. At first he didn't much like it, finding it hard work, but I tried to show him that riding a mountain bike properly was just like driving a performance car, changing up and down through the gears for the best results. Well that made sense to Colin and suddenly he understood and then got interested in the technical aspects of the sport. Cycling has become as much a part of Colin's work as testing the car, and everywhere he goes there's a Scott mountain bike in the motorhome. By getting Colin fit on a bike, the biggest thing he gained was the endurance to push himself through the later stages of

Mark Webber digs deep on the Tasmanian challenge

long days behind the wheel while under intense pressure – especially when conditions in the cockpit of a rally car can reach concentration-sapping temperatures of more than 50°C. The cycle training gave him the additional endurance, which meant he could focus on his driving, not on his aching muscles. These days Colin acknowledges that his improved fitness has given him the extra edge he needs when competing against the best in the world.

When he had a huge accident during the rally of Corsica in 2000, Colin was about a quarter of an hour away from death after hanging upside down in his car for 45 minutes. He is very lucky to be alive and probably the main thing that kept him alive during the aftermath of the accident was his conditioning. Being fit helped save Colin's life – and cycling had played an important part in getting him fit.

WHAT DO YOU WEAR ON A BIKE?

'Aye, there's the rub', as Shakespeare said. Proper padded cycle shorts will protect you from sores and a pain where you really don't want them and use chammy cream – available from any good bike shop. In winter, long thermal leggings are a must and you can also get thermal arm warmers, which are useful because you can take them off (they fit into your back pocket) once you've warmed up.

On the top, you need a proper thermal type of vest that wicks away the sweat. Wearing technologically-developed cycle tops is not just about fashion. Cycling is unusual in that your body can often experience sudden extremes of

Safety and equipment

So cycling is a fantastic low-impact aerobic activity with the added advantage that it can take you out into the great outdoors, allowing you to explore wonderful new environments, but first things first. Cycling does have certain risks attached to it, not the least of which are other road users and there are no excuses for not sorting out your personal safety before you set off on your ride.

- If you have bought a new bike then make sure you take it back to the dealer after the second or so ride. Get it checked over (we call this a spanner check), as parts that have just experienced their first real movement and weight bearing will start to loosen off.
- Make sure you have good tyre pressure – for road bikes you want about 95psi roughly, for mountain bikes about 40–50psi depending on whether you are riding hard-packed trails or soft terrain.
- Get a good quality helmet straight away (I absolutely refuse to take anyone out on a ride without a helmet from a recognised manufacturer – no helmet, no ride!).
- Make sure you have a toolkit, which fits underneath the saddle, that has two spare inner tubes, a small toolkit with alum keys and a couple of tyre levers.
- You must have a bottle cage to put a bottle of fluids in and an attachment for a pump. Do not go out without a pump – ever. If you do, especially in remote rural areas, you are in for a long, slow and painful walk home!

temperature. You can be tackling a long sweaty climb then turn a corner and suddenly be facing straight into a gusting wind or, after reaching the summit of the climb, you start a rapid descent which doesn't require anything like the same physical effort and has a wind chill factor as well. And in both cases you will get totally chilled – so you need specially designed clothing that will wick away moisture from the skin. I always carry a lightweight nylon windcheater-type top as well, so as soon as I know it's getting a bit chilly I will stop quickly and put that on.

Always wear proper cycle gloves. Normally they're fingerless, but in the winter you need to change to a thermal-type glove. Now, during training camps, I'm responsible for the safety and continuing health of some very expensive athletes (particularly F1 drivers), and I can tell you that none of them get on a bike without cycle gloves – for a very simple reason. What's the first thing that is going to come into contact with the hard, unforgiving road or gritty track or path when you fall off? Yes, your delicate hands, and the gravel is going to get into your torn-up palms. You will be astonished at how long it takes for that sort of wound to heal.

EQUIPMENT SET-UP

I always recommend spending time getting the set-up of your bike right before doing any work. It's easy to forget to do this in the gym: you jump onto the exercise bike and pedal away as if your life depended on it. If the seat is set too high, you may find you develop hip problems and if you hyper-extend your

knee it can lead to problems at the back of the knee. On the other hand, if the seat is set too low, then you may experience problems with the patella tendon.

To set yourself correctly, sit on the bike with your hips nice and square, and the heel of your foot – in your training shoe – on the pedal at its lowest point. Your leg should be soft, not completely straight, so that when the ball of your foot is on the pedal, you can see a slight angle.

There is a formula for working this out (this is based on the assumption you are using standard 172.5mm road cranks). Stand with your feet, in socks not training shoes this time, the width of the crank on the cycle, and then take a measurement from your groin straight down to the floor. Multiply that distance by 0.885 and you'll get the ideal distance from the top of the saddle to the middle of the crank. This is called the Hinault formula, named after the great Bernard Hinault, one of the all-time great Tour de France champions.

For me the groin to floor height is 89.5cm, so multiplied by 0.885 I get an ideal distance of 79cm – you can adjust this a centimetre either way. Pro cycle shops have a jig to measure this perfect set-up.

I also want to add a word about something that can put you off cycling if you haven't got it right when you first start out or when you climb back on a bike after a considerable layoff. If you are going to buy a new bike make sure you get advice on saddles. These days you will find that there are a number of types of gel saddles available, but be aware that too much of a padded saddle can create its own

Nothing can beat fresh mountain air. Ride your bike with body and machine in harmony.

problems. Basically there are two things you can do: either buy a gel padded cover (which can easily be removed at a later date) or try to get used to the effects of sitting on a bike by conditioning – i.e. take shorter rides at first and expect to feel as if you are bit bruised around the coccyx. As you gradually progress with regular rides, you will find that the problem of an aching rear end will disappear.

GEAR RATIOS IN CYCLING

How many of you know what size chain rings and sprockets you've got on your bike? Most competitive racers will, but even some of them won't. This has always amazed me as it is a crucial performance factor in racing and in making cycling more efficient and enjoyable in general.

Gear ratios allow the rider to adjust the mechanical advantage of the drive system on a bike. In a low gear, the pedals turn really easily, but you have to pedal much faster (i.e. with higher rpm) to get significant speed up; these are the gears you use to go uphill. In a high gear, the pedals are harder to turn, but you don't have to pedal them round as quickly to make the bike go as fast.

The speed at which you push the pedals around is referred to as cadence and using the right gear to get the optimum cadence is vital for racing cyclists, who, while going as fast as possible, need to conserve as much energy as they can. They also need the leg speed and flexibility to deal with the sudden changes of pace that occur in racing. For the rest of us, whatever the

level of our performance, it's just as important – you need to get the most from your efforts without getting heavy legs or riding inefficiently.

Producing the optimum cadence will depend on a lot of factors. Well-trained professional riders will often 'spin' along at 100rpm with minimum loading per revolution, even at relatively high speeds, to save their legs for any sprints, climbs or attacks later in a race. This is an efficient cadence for them because of the hours of training they have spent perfecting the technique, but for a beginner spinning at 100rpm would feel uncoordinated and out of control, so 80 or so rpm might be more comfortable. Downhill or on the flat a higher optimum cadence is often used compared with climbing. There are riders (the most famous of all being Lance Armstrong) who spin very fast – up to 115 rpm – for extended periods and find this very effective. Other riders, however, particularly in time trialling might prefer to 'roll' a big gear much more slowly but with a high power output per revolution.

Bikes these days are sophisticated pieces of equipment and the number of gears available on most machines can be quite considerable and their set-up quite a technical issue. The ratio between the gears of any given machine can be set up in two ways – either to give the rider a wide spread of gears or, alternatively, a number of narrowly grouped gears. Most mountain bikes rely on a wide spread of gears to cope with the huge variety of steep and difficult hills, whereas road bikes, ridden on terrain which is less extreme, are set up with very 'close ratio' gears that allow the rider to find his or her optimum cadence on a given gradient or at a given pace, which in turn produces the best economy of effort.

Do you know what 53 x 12 means? It refers to the number of teeth on the big front chain ring where the cranks are attached times the number of teeth on the rear sprocket on the back wheel of the bike. To be able to compare various combinations of gearing, a method of measurement in 'inches' is used. This has been around for years and was really important in my dad's day (see the picture on page 8) when you only had one gear in a fixed wheel – so getting it right before you set off was important! These days you don't hear about fixed wheels, except on the track where they are still used. We're now a bit spoilt, with as many as 30 gears on a road bike (some have a triple chain ring on the front and 10-speed block at the back).

CYCLING TECHNIQUE: DEVELOPING FLEXIBILITY IN THE ANKLES

To get the most out of your cycling you need to work on turning the pedals properly. That probably sounds obvious or too simple. But you'd be amazed at how many people ignore this key part of cycling. It's very easy to get hung up on the machinery and forget about the basics. Cycling is not just a matter of pushing the pedals round as hard as possible.

What you should be aiming to achieve is the most efficient and economical use of your quads – the four major muscles of the front of the leg – and the hamstring, which pulls your leg, and the pedal, back up.

Using the flexbility in your ankles to

produce a smooth elliptical movement is the correct motion which is called the souplesse.

If you're out on your bike try out the principles first of all on a flat piece of road. Later, once you feel comfortable with the technique, try going downhill and taking one foot out of the toe clips or off the pedal, so you can concentrate on one ankle at a time. If your bottom bracket is clunking, you're probably not ankling correctly.

If you're in the gym, try to use a bike trainer rather than an exercise bike, otherwise you'll be fighting against its inbuilt electric braking system.

Turn the pedals at between 85 and 90rpm and, if you can, use a mirror to watch your technique. If you find yourself bobbing up and down, you're pressing on the pedals too hard. Relax, and try dropping the loading.

CYCLING TECHNIQUE: SUSPENSION, BALANCE AND BRAKING

When you head down to your local mountain bike shop and spend your money on your new bike it will have either no suspension, front suspension or dual suspension (which means front and rear suspension for use, mainly, on extreme off-road). That said I like it because it stops all the stresses going through the lower back while the youngsters, with their good conditioned backs, can deal with it. I recommend that anyone who is planning to go off-road should buy a bike with front suspension that will soak up a lot of the stress that will otherwise go through their forearms.

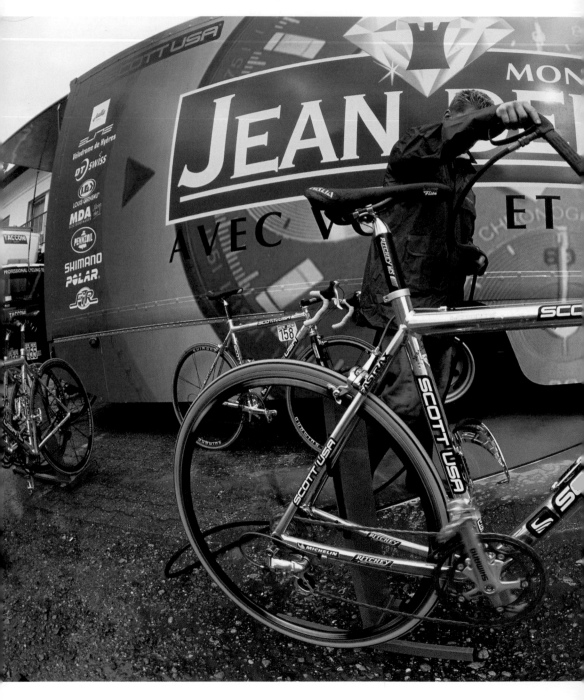

Tour de France: when you race at this level you even get someone to wash your bike!

Bernie's tip
Work on higher cadences (95–100rpm) rather than pushing a big gear to improve your cycling.

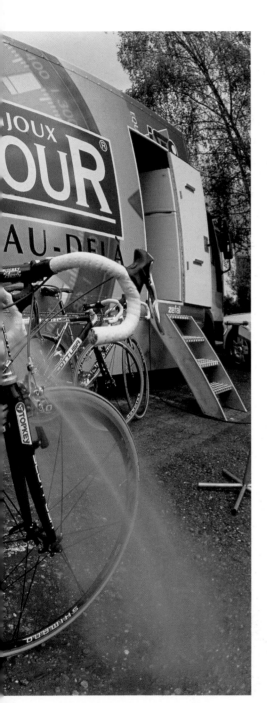

When you are descending hillsides at speed there are a couple of simple things I recommend you to do: make sure the chain is in the middle chain ring out of the three at the front and that you have the pedals parallel to the floor – don't have one pedal up and one down. It's easy for a rock to catch underneath your lower pedal and throw you off the bike. And because you will be in a stood-up type of position, make certain you are actually pinching the saddle with the inner part of your thighs. The reason for this is simple and a lesson you will only want to learn once: if you are 'loose' on the bike and do hit a bump, you can fall off and if you get your anatomy wrapped round the crossbar there will be plenty of tears before bedtime.

Another thing is to think about the way you brake on a bike. Just as you wouldn't brake late and heavily when cornering in a car, well it's the same on a bike because the back will flip around just as easily, and then you'll be in that rose bush before you know it. Look ahead and anticipate your braking point and try to assess the conditions of the road surface or terrain. Unlike a car, however, you do have to think about the balance between front and back wheel braking. Too hard on the back brake and you are likely to lock out the back wheel which means a skid, and obviously you don't want to hit the front brake too hard or you will end up over the handlebar. It is all about having control. Brake early and get the speed out of the corners rather than brake harshly, make errors and lose lots of time or upset your ride with a crash.

Buying a bike

If you are new to cycling you could easily be forgiven for being thoroughly confused by the huge variety of bikes on offer, so before you rush off and buy your new bike begin by asking yourself what sort of cycling you want to take up. Think about the likely locations you plan to ride and the sort of terrains you will want to ride on, and just why you have decided to give this wonderful sport (and, let's not forget, mode of transport) a go. Then visit a professional bike shop that will advise you appropriately. Once you've made your choice they'll set up you and your new bike properly and safely (don't forget the helmet!). Here are some examples of types of bikes to help you make up your mind.

1. Beginners/children's mountain bike: basic entry level bike for learning to ride and short distance leisure riding. Styled like a mountain bike, some may even have front suspension forks and treaded tyres but are not suitable for serious off-roading. They would be fine for towpaths and other good off-road surfaces.

2. Leisure/freeride mountain bike: more advanced bike for general off- and on-road use. Lighter weight and full suspension. Suitable for more adventurous off-road riding with the right tyres and suspension settings.

3. Downhill mountain bike: specialist competition bike for downhill racers. These bikes tend to have much greater suspension travel to soak up big hits at high speed. Made heavier and stronger than cross-country bikes as the riders don't have to ride them up the hills as well. Often they have bigger gear ratios and more powerful disc brakes to deal with higher speeds.

4. Rigid cross-country mountain bike: designed to be fast up and downhill over all terrains. Often with front suspension to take some of the vibrations and bumps out of the track. Can also be used with slick tyres on the road if you have only one bike for training and competing. These are the most popular choice for most leisure riders off- and on-road because they deal well with all conditions, including bumping up and down curbs in town, and can cope equally well with a ride in the woods, a trip to the shops or a race in a mountain bike competition.

5. Road racing bike: a specialist bike made to be very light and rigid for maximum speed on the road. Variations on the design are used for all forms of road riding from touring to time trialling and road racing. Very fast and efficient on the tarmac, these bikes are totally unsuitable for any kind of off-road riding and so are aimed at a more specialist market.

Bernie's tip
When you are buying a new bike don't be swayed by pretty colours: always invest in the quality of the moving components – e.g. the wheels and the chain set.

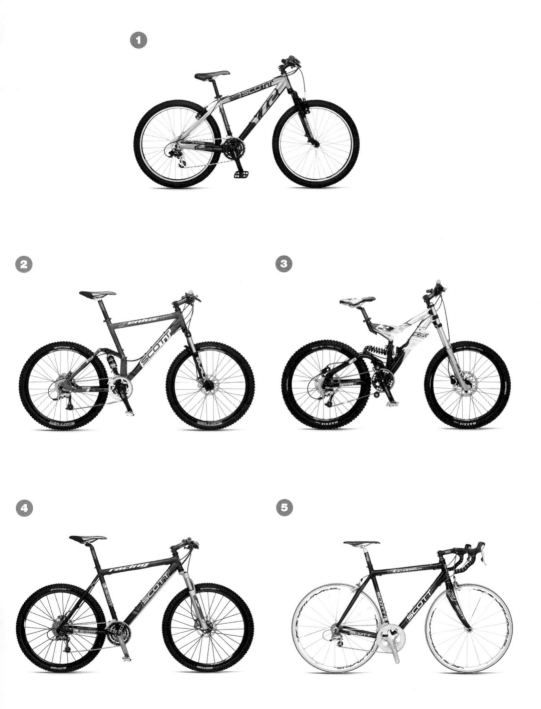

Swimming

ALTHOUGH I HAVE ALWAYS ENJOYED taking part in all water-based sports – especially canoeing and surfing – I only began to get seriously involved in swimming in my 20s as part of the triathlon discipline. When I started swimming I soon realised the importance of mastering good swimming technique; and later on I made sure that my kids got into swimming at an early age.

To work your way through this challenging element, you need to develop a 'feel for the water': anyone who's watched Ian Thorpe competing during the Olympics or Commonwealth Games will have seen how he makes it seem so effortless, as if he is in perfect harmony with the water, so much so that some other world-class competitors look awkward in comparison.

The best way to learn about swimming is to get in there and do it; it's a bit like golf. You can read about technique and

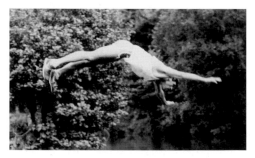

Diving into just half a metre of water during *Survival of the Fittest* in 1987. I had to judge this just right

look at all the photographs and diagrams till the cows come home, but there is no substitute for getting in the water and doing the real thing; and when your stroke (in both sports) is in the groove, it feels fantastic. But no matter what level of swimming you are at, the basic fundamentals of body position – leg action, arm action, breathing and timing of the swim stroke – apply to everyone. At all levels (leisure as well as competitive swimming) I see the difficulties that arise when swimmers try too hard, racing quickly in order to either keep up or get ahead. Rushing the swim stroke in an attempt to go faster is often the root of all technique-related problems. Swimming without control over the basic elements leads to excessive fatigue and resistance, and ultimately frustration.

If you are looking to improve your swimming performances, then start by learning to swim slower with more control. In competition, experienced and elite swimmers will have a stroke rate of between 70 and 120 strokes per minute (approximately) depending on the event, which equals between one and two strokes every second. By slowing this rate down by at least 50% when working on technique, you will find that you have more time to control your actions.

Physiotherapists have always highlighted the value of swimming and hydrotherapy movements in the water for

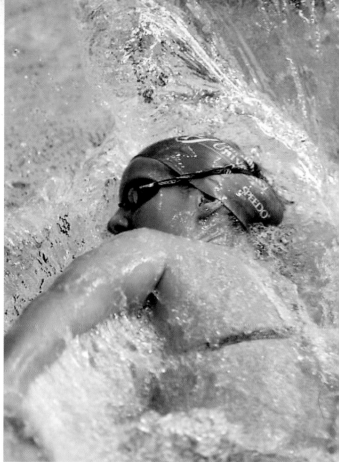

remedial and rehabilitation benefits following injury. Once I started training for triathlon, I found that the number of injuries I was incurring in my other sporting activities was considerably reduced; swimming really is a great sport for total body conditioning. The action provides good blood flow to all your muscles and, quite simply, it keeps you ticking over. That is why I always get in the pool the day after a hard race to ease my muscles off and enhance recovery.

As swimming is a non-weight-bearing activity it's an ideal sport once your joints start to complain. As you get older (and I include myself in this category these days) you must be aware of not overstressing your joints as they won't stand up to the sort of loading they did when you were in your 20s. So if you are no longer in the spring chicken category, make sure you're not spending too much time sitting down. Get out and get active; and swimming is one of the best activities, whatever your age.

Once your basic swimming technique is in place, you can use swimming as an endurance training activity, either swimming continuously or in structured sets. If you find this boring, then you can break down the training session into phases. On pages 60 and 61 Robin Brew, former Olympic record holder for the 200m and these days a top swimming coach, has put together a series of training sessions for you to try. They are based on:

1 The warm-up
2 Drills concentrating on technique
3 Building up longer intervals at a steady pace
4 Sprints
5 The cool down

When competing actively I have always benefited from this kind of thought-through mix more than the full-on, overintense training that some swimming clubs lean towards. In the United Kingdom, British swimming is definitely on the up and the widely acclaimed Long Term Athlete Plan (LTAP) that has been written by the Amateur Swimming Association is designed to safeguard the interests of our youngsters, ensuring that there is gradual, goal-oriented progression – based on age, gender and physical development. Gone are the days

A perfect example of good breathing technique – note the bow wave (see page 59)

Swimming is the cheapest form of physiotherapy you can get, as long as you can swim.

when young club swimmers were pushed very hard and very early. Unfortunately a culture of pushing too hard, too early still exists in other sports and a 'train for the session' rather than 'train for the goal' attitude is, I think, detrimental.

Swimmers just wanting to keep fit often ignore the importance of technique. It's well worth getting some lessons from a qualified coach or swimming teacher, who will assess your technique and give you feedback and advice on how to improve it. This will save you hours of poor swimming, and will fast track your improvement, making your time in the water more interesting, challenging and exciting.

As far as the different strokes are concerned, I would generally concentrate on combining breaststroke, freestyle and backstroke. Butterfly is certainly a very challenging technical stroke which requires good timing of the leg and arm action to be performed well. Don't discount this wonderful stroke – you can have a lot of fun practising it over short distances of between 10 and 15 metres.

I will generally use a float when practising my leg kick on my front, however you can kick on your back or on either side of the body when using a frontcrawl, backstroke or butterfly leg action. Kicking without a board is a great way to improve core stability and lower back strength – perfect for F1 racing drivers.

To learn correct technique as an adult, if you had no training when you were young, requires real application and a commitment to attend some serious instructional courses. A coach on the poolside can help you both to improve

your stroke efficiency and also develop a better feel for the water. The feedback and corrections that a good coach can provide are invaluable if you are looking to make a significant improvement to your swimming in a short period of time. Remember swimming is one of those sports that is difficult to self-analyse or determine on your own exactly what you are doing wrong. You can't really use a mirror in a swimming pool!

Even if you only want to swim to keep fit, or because the last time you had any training was lining up along the poolside at school, I do recommend that you seek out professional coaching. This is one sport where you really cannot afford to pick up bad habits. A few sessions will give you the basic fundamentals of swimming efficiency, and the basic principles of the swim stroke. If you are prepared to put in the effort, you will reap the rewards; swimming is a great sport for giving you all-round conditioning, utilising the majority of the primary muscle groups, with minimal weight bearing involved, as well as giving your cardiovascular system an excellent workout.

For the leisure swimmer, I generally prefer people to mix their strokes which will have the benefit of conditioning different muscle groups. Be careful with the kicking action of the breaststroke: snapping it out too aggressively can lead to injury. But that doesn't mean you shouldn't do the breaststroke; if you feel comfortable with it, mix the stroke up with freestyle, backstroke and some work kicking while holding a float.

Although I am not going to try to write a

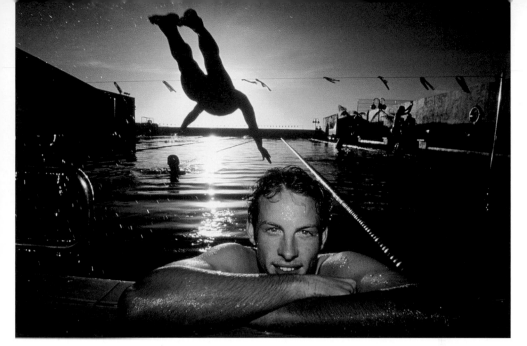

swimming manual, or replace any formal lessons, here are a few thoughts to bear in mind when you are swimming – but this really is only the tip of the iceberg, a few principles to get you started.

In a nutshell, to move forward in swimming you have to apply backward pressure with the arms. If the pressure applied is in the wrong direction then opposite forces occur creating resistance and drag. To help create an image that might be useful, imagine you are a rower in a single scull (if you have ever tried to row one you will know what I am on about!). Balance is everything; one wrong move and you are in the water. The idea is to sit tall and still, the movements of the stroke include, just like swimming, a catch phase, a sweep stroke and an exit and recovery. Now imagine if the rower pulled too deep with one blade. The scull would keel over to that side causing loss of balance, rhythm, timing and ultimately speed, not to mention the extra effort required to recover from the fault. To row well requires a great deal of discipline; a lot of time is spent developing balance and timing at slower speeds so that when

the pace is gradually increased, the control and efficiency of the stroke remains. This is exactly the same principle required to develop a more effective swimming stroke. The reason all this is so often overlooked is, by and large, lack of confidence and understanding. The need to keep up and try to swim fast must not overshadow the learning of key skills. Speed will come as you improve your swimming efficiency.

If you haven't been involved with swimming for a while, get used to simply floating. Once in the water, relax, lie on your back and acquire a sense of your natural buoyancy. Some people have very strong positive buoyancy; others will find themselves sinking automatically, in other words they have negative buoyancy. This is due to your personal mix of bone/ muscle density. If you find your buoyancy is negative it does not mean you cannot swim, since swimming is all about propulsion – if you are negatively buoyant you will just have to expend more effort.

The goal in your head should be to remain relaxed and streamlined. We've all experienced that moment in the holiday

Jenson takes a rest. I take a dive

If you are splashing like a drowning cow, that's efficiently and try to progress in the water with

hotel pool when your brain is telling you that you look like a slimline torpedo, and everybody else thinks you look like a washing machine.

In the freestyle stroke, you are pulling your body over your hand in the water, so the image you should have is of holding the water; imagine you are holding a beachball out in front of you, then picture a tray of sand, and scoop your hand back through the tray of sand along your body's centreline. Another way to think about it is to visualise a rope running underneath the centre of your body, and that there is a series of pockets along the rope that you have to put your hand into to pull yourself along.

If you are splashing like a drowning cow, that's a sure sign that you are fighting the water. Work efficiently and try to progress in the water with fewer rather than more strokes.

A good way to build up the necessary gliding profile is to push off from the side, with your hands in front of you, locked straight out. Enjoy the gliding sensation and see where you have got to each time – the further the better. This should help you to feel streamlined and relaxed when you are actually swimming.

Try swimming short distances from a push-off, say 6–10 slow strokes without breathing (this is called hypoxic training). Repeat this over and over again until you can sense a high body position and a smooth, relaxed, rhythmical arm action. The key is to work on the overall body relaxation while keeping the shoulders, hips and heels high and in line with the surface of the water. Use a relaxed, shallow, gentle leg action to assist.

The breathing cycle when performed incorrectly is the biggest disruption to the balance of the body and all the key components of the stroke: it accounts for the majority of problems experienced by novice and improving swimmers. Sometimes breathing problems arise out of a fear of the water and it's not unusual to see swimmers holding their breath for several strokes then quickly grabbing a lungful of air in an awkward head-twisting movement. Think about it: would you hold your breath for any length of time if you were out jogging? Learn to breathe out slowly into the water (this is called trickle

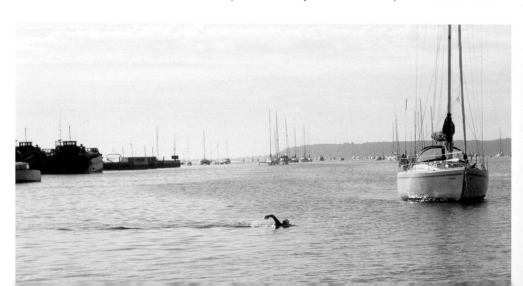

a sure sign that you are fighting the water. Work fewer rather than more strokes.

breathing) and then inhale as your head rises naturally out of the water as part of the stroke: your forward movement will generate a bow wave, behind which will be the trough that you use to take your breath without lifting the head. See the picture on page 55.

To practise fitting the breathing movements into the stroke, stand in the shallow end leaning forward with your shoulders submerged below the surface and one arm extended with the other arm by your side. Take a breath and place your head into the water. With the leading hand remaining still and extended, begin to exhale fully, turning your head 90 degrees to the side as you near the completion of your exhalation. Now begin your inhalation, taking a good clear breath before turning your head back to the centre line. This should be repeated over and over again until the timing seems to become easier and the movements of the head are smooth. It may be useful to stand with one leg forward and one leg backward as this can simulate the natural roll of the body.

The main thing to understand about the breathing cycle is that the breathing fits into the framework of the stroke. Therefore, whether you breathe or not, the stroke movements always remain the same.

The leg kick message is, once again, relax. If your ankles are too stiff you won't make any progress. In fact I've seen some cyclists working in the pool whose ankles are so stiff they end up going backwards... Try swimming with your toes pulled towards your shins and you'll see what I mean. Point your toes for

Ocean swimming: If you want to swim in the sea, a special swimming wetsuit is a very good idea to make sure your body stays at an acceptable temperature. There are a huge number of people who prefer to swim in the sea without a wetsuit all year round (and hats off to them I say). A wetsuit, however, will give you greater buoyancy – which means that you will use your arms more and your legs less, helping to develop your shoulder strength.

maximum forward movement.

Finally, give yourself a structure for a swimming session, as you would for any training session. Don't jump in and plough up and down for 30 lengths and then towel down. Include a warm-up, a conditioning phase and a cool down. You hear about top-level swimmers knocking out 7km sessions (that's 280 lengths to you and me), but they achieve that by breaking the session down into achievable goals. So you can do the same: just swimming up and down the pool, week in week out, will leave you brain-dead and your motivation will drop off. Remember what I said earlier: train for the goal not for the session.

Bernie's tip
The older we get the more we should take to the water to increase mobility of the joints and to condition the majority of the muscle groups.

Andy Blow swimming against a 4-knot tide in Poole harbour

An advanced swimming programme

Robin Brew (former Olympic record holder for the 200 metre individual medley and 4 times world record holder)

EVEN BEFORE THE MERITS OF FITNESS and conditioning are discussed, learning to swim well is essential. From a personal survival point of view we want to be safe and confident in the water, where so much enjoyment and fun can be had. Swimming well opens up many, many possibilities from surfing to scuba diving, from water polo to water skiing. To simply play on the waves at the beach can leave you with a sense of exhilaration.

Swimming, therefore, is undoubtedly one of the best all-round exercises for people of all ages and, what's more, both technique and fitness can be developed and improved at any age. Swimming forms an essential part of any cross-training programme and whether you are a triathlete or a keen fitness swimmer then learning the frontcrawl is a must, as it is the fastest of all the four individual strokes. It is also the stroke that is swum the most in training and racing by competitive swimmers because of its conditioning benefits.

Learning the frontcrawl need not be complicated if the basic principles are understood. The stroke requires balance and coordination, a little like riding a bike. In its simplest form, the frontcrawl stroke can be broken down into five parts:
1 Body position, 2 Leg action, 3 Arm action, 4 Breathing and 5 Timing

The timing of the stroke must coordinate and link each component together and will dictate how effective and smooth the stroke becomes. The coordination of the stroke is, from the start, more important than the application of effort and force delivered through the arm and leg action.

By and large, the movements that are made in all swimming strokes conform to Newton's third law of motion – 'an action creates an equally opposite reaction'. Therefore if you do something wrong on one side of the stroke, you are sure enough going to have a counter problem on the other side. A simple example: if you incorrectly press down to assist the breathing and lift your head high, then your legs at the other end of the body are going to sink.

The key to getting the swimming stroke right is to make the least possible disruption to the balance, forward propulsion and streamlining of the stroke. By aiming to swim with a smooth, relaxed, rhythmical arm action the stroke will be more effective and ultimately efficient.

Here are a few simple examples of training sessions for you to try in order of intensity.

To keep a check on your progress and to keep you motivated, aim to swim a straight 400m timed against the clock every 4 to 5 weeks. See if you can gradually work your time down to under 8 minutes. If you are recording between 7 and 8 minutes for your 400m then that is very encouraging. If you are swimming between 6 and 7 minutes you are swimming at a good pace. Between 5 and 6 minutes you would be able to keep up with most masters swimming club sessions. Between 4 and 5 minutes you would be very competitive in most local competitions and less than 4 minutes give me a call! The world record is currently held by Ian Thorpe and stands at an incredible 3 minutes 40 seconds.

1. Aerobic and technique session I (low–moderate intensity)	2. Aerobic and technique session II (low–moderate intensity)	3. Anaerobic threshold session (moderate–high intensity)	4. Speed work (sprints)	5. VO₂ Max session (very high intensity)
Warm-up *Repeat twice* 150m f/c breathe every third stroke 50m f/c kick with kick board	**Warm-up** 200m f/c 100m f/c kick with kick board 200m pull (arms only using a float)	**Warm-up** 400m f/c or 100m f/c plus 100m catch up (one single arm stroke then the other)	**Warm-up** 300m f/c every third 25m single arm 100m leg kick on side (one arm forward, one arm by side) change side every 25m 200m alternate f/c and backstroke every 50m	**Warm-up** 200m f/c – breathe every third or fourth arm stroke 4 x 50m as 25m f/c plus 25m any other stroke than f/c with 30 second RI
Build set 4 x 50m f/c increase speed but maintain stroke count each 50m with 30 second RI	**Build set** *Repeat twice* 100m f/c Pull – build each 100m to a fast last 15m with 45 second RI	**Build set** 4 x 25m f/c kick increase speed each 25m with 20 second RI 4 x 25m swim increase speed each 25m with 20 second RI	**Build set** 4 x 25m f/c – increase speed into a sprint over the last 10m with 45 second RI	**Build set** 3 x 50m f/c kick – increase speed each 50m with 30 second RI
Main set 2 x 50m f/c drills (single arm with other arm extended) with 20 second RI 200m f/c low intensity but good technique and turns with 30 second RI 2 x 50m f/c drills (single arm with other arm by side) with 20 second RI 200m f/c low intensity but good technique and turns with 30 second RI 2 x 50m f/c drills (catch up – one single arm stroke then the other) with 20 second RI 200m f/c moderate intensity but good technique and turns with 30 second RI	**Main set** *Repeat twice* 500m f/c with 2 minutes RI **1** Aim to maintain distance per stroke and rhythm **2** Try to maintain an even pace **3** Heart rate should be approximately 40bpm below your maximum **4** Make the time for both 500m as close as possible	**Main set** 20 to 30 x 25m swim with 10 second RI Aim to hold the fastest even pace possible throughout the whole set	**Main set** 10 x 50m with 60 seconds between each 50m as: **1** 15m fast + 35m easy **2** 25m fast + 25m easy **3** 35m fast + 15m easy **4** 50m fast **5** 50m recovery *Repeat twice*	**Main set** 75m f/c then a 30 second RI 50m f/c then a 30 second RI 25m f/c then a 30 second RI Increase speed and effort from 75m – 25m and also make each set faster No extra rest between sets *Repeat set 4 times*
Swim down 200m any other stroke	**Swim down** 4 x 50m easy mixing strokes with 20 second RI	**Swim down** 300m easy – choice of strokes	**Swim down** 8 x 50m – mixing strokes, easy with 15 second RI	**Swim down** 300m easy – choice of strokes
Total 1500m	**Total 1900m**	**Total 1400–1650m**	**Total 1600m**	**Total 1150m**

key: f/c frontcrawl, RI rest interval

Kayaking

WATER IS AN INCREDIBLE ELEMENT.
Fill up a kayak with water and you won't be
able to pick it up. But get that same kayak
on top of some white water and it will
move like magic as you are suddenly
thrown into dynamic motion, trying not to
battle with the forces unleashed by a
raging river, but working with them to make
your way down or upstream in this
exhilarating challenge. Of course, you don't
need to be on an extreme torrent to be
able to enjoy kayaking.

Like all the sporting activities I tend to
favour, kayaking is another that will get
you outdoors and appreciating the natural
environment. I spend a lot of time on the
River Stour at Canford Magna in Dorset:
first thing in the morning, with the mist
hovering over the river, trees all along the
banks – it's sheer pleasure. A great
holiday is descending the Ardèche river in
France which offers superb paddling and
scenery, and I thoroughly enjoy going for a
15-mile paddle down the Wye Valley with
my son Gregg.

Kayaking was one of my first loves, and
one which helped me begin to take sport
seriously. This was mainly due to the initial
encouragement I received from one of my
school teachers, Laurie Porter, who
organised the canoe classes at my school
on a lake (actually a large pond) about five
miles from the school.

Laurie was brilliant with an attention to
detail about every element of technique

that was phenomenal: it's stayed with me
to this day. He took me on my first Grade
Three paddle at Symond's Yat in the West
Country. Here I found real excitement,
paddling in white water for the first time.
Laurie's great strength was the way he
would describe the river so that you
formed a vivid mental map which meant
you could read the river accurately once
you were on it – it wasn't academic
theory, but real practical information
based on his enormous experience.

It was the recruitment advert showing two
Royal Marines in canoes that got me
interested in the corps. Of course, as it
turned out, I never saw a bloody canoe for
two and a half years, and the only water I
came into contact with was when we had to
cross rivers and then it was always freezing,
but I still kept my enthusiasm for the sport...!

In the past few years I've been doing
more and more kayaking, changing over
to K1 paddling. An aspect of the sport
about which I have become particularly
aware is the role of balance in kayaking;
the craft is very unstable, so you really do
have to develop a sense of balance or you
are going to get very wet very quickly.

Once your balance and technique is in
place, you need to develop what I call a
'feel for water', just as you have to do in
swimming. Your blade becomes an
extension of yourself, your lever to work
with the water, using its own forces to
achieve what you want to do. This is not

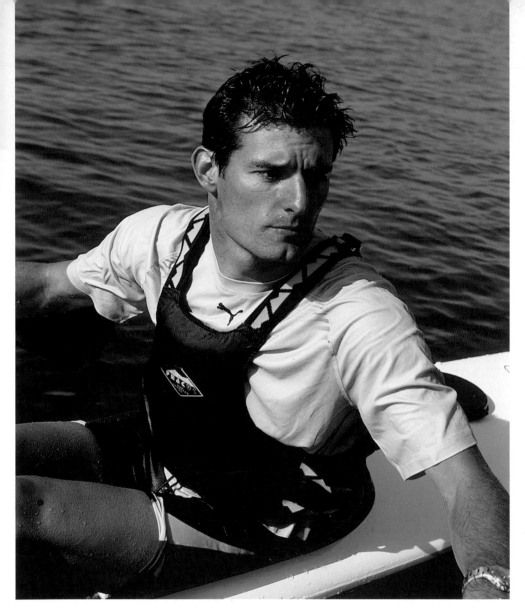

just about strength, either; watch the top women kayakers dancing round the rocks and slabs in their way in a slalom event and you'll quickly realise that brute force is far less important than a level of real technical skill and balance.

I once went on a Grade Five stretch of white water of the Durance near Briançon with Rick Grice: this was extreme white water. We spent two hours studying each element of a stretch of river only 800 metres long, so that we knew exactly what the water was doing at each stage.

At this extreme end you can taste your own fear – even when you know that all along the rocks on the banks are safety teams watching out for you. Originally the water made me scared, but I learnt to overcome the fear and to enjoy the adrenalin rush that accompanies resisting a river's attempts to throw you against a rock face.

Whichever form of canoeing you get involved in, you'll enjoy the thrill of coping with the challenges that the water gives

Stay upright! Mark Webber has just learnt the importance of balance in a canoe

you. One of my particular favourites is the 'stopper', where the river drops and the flow rate is high. You can sit on a stopper, and then suddenly the water will pop your nose down and spit you right out. What a rush – that's my kind of sport!

I've already briefly mentioned Alexander Popov, the top Russian freestyle swimmer. Popov used K1 paddling mechanics and technique to better understand and improve his frontcrawl stroke. I really am in favour of going to the next level and getting swimmers in a K1 some of the time to get away from the black line of the pool and out on the river for a change. I have found I can still swim pretty well these days even though I'm rarely motivated to get in the pool and it's the paddling that has given me that ability. The only thing I feel I lack now is a feel for the water in the hands and in the arms that only comes from hours spent in the pool.

Essentially I am in my second season of serious marathon paddling at the moment. Looking back to the time when I was a cross-country skier, I wish I had known more about the biomechanics of paddling because these days it obviously delivers real benefits in upper body work and core stability. In fact, there are not many endurance sports it will not complement in some way or another.

Within the overall sport of canoeing there are various groups of activities, and kayaking is one of the most diverse, more than most people realise. I suppose you could compare it to running in that you can be a sprinter (like a track athlete) all the way through to an out-and-out endurance specialist doing the DW, which is the paddling equivalent of a tough fell race.

K1 and K2: K1 (one person craft) and K2 (two person craft) race in competitions ranging from sprinting 1000m up to DW (125 miles). Sprinting is done in lanes on a rowing lake and the marathon takes place on rivers and canals, often involving portages (where you have to carry the craft over a lock gate or weir), a significant part of the longer races that requires some specific training.

The craft are high volume, low resistance, which means they are very fast but very unstable on the water. When I first started out in a K1, with my background of paddling white water and surf, I simply couldn't believe the balance required to just sit in the thing (I had a top-end racing craft). Even after being the passenger in a K2 I thought it would be a natural transition. Wrong. I spent a lot of time getting wet and honestly thought my boat was defective. It got to the stage where I thought that a sport I loved was going to defeat me, but good advice and a lot of practice in the early hours of the morning over the winter gradually paid off and I now put it in the same category as cross-country skiing as a remarkable, graceful sport.

When I did get the balance sorted out I needed to learn the best technique to maximise performance. Using a wing paddle was challenging because the mechanics require a rotation of the trunk, pivoting from the hips. To maximise the efficiency of the boat as the blade enters the water, the foot on that same side drives into the footrest to lock out the hip

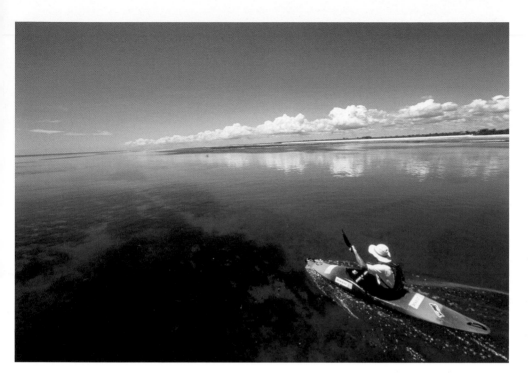

region; the trunk then rotates with the arms held almost statically so that the power for the stroke comes from the rotation of the upper body. The way this has best been described to me is that you drive the paddle into the water as if it were a stake that you then pull yourself past, as if on rollerskates. This process repeats in a cycle – and actually cycling is one way to describe the leg action as you press from one leg to the other as the blade enters the water on either side.

If ever there were two sports that could deliver all-round fitness – forever – they would be cross-country skiing and K1 paddling. It's a great pity that they're both such minority sports. Physically I get huge returns in the hip region from the cycling leg motion, in my trunk, core, all over the back and to a degree in my legs.

Any kind of fitness benefits that come with doing a specific sport will obviously complement other sports, but I think that K1 has an edge on many with its unique combination of skill factors, its requirement for good back strength, balance and upper body work. My cycling has certainly been enhanced (especially sitting in on the climbs) by the driving of the legs in paddling, as has running uphill – even though I'm only doing these sports occasionally these days.

Slalom: for this type of paddling the boats are lower volume, easier to manoeuvre and relatively more stable than a K1. The competitive elements of the sport involve being timed over a course of up to about two minutes in duration with gates to negotiate both upstream and downstream. It requires speed and accuracy in placing the boat between the gates. The gates are often placed on difficult sections such as a stopper wave or boiler to test the competitor's skills to the full. This is where I had my first real outings in competitive sport by entering slalom races when I was about thirteen years old.

Sometimes a canoe can take you to a very special place

Kayak comparison chart

K1 marathon 12 miles+	Slalom – fast-flowing water
Endurance activity 60 min + events	Highly anaerobic 1–3 min event
Flat water	White water
Constant rhythm of paddling	Explosive and reactive to water conditions
Category mass start racing	Time trial against the clock
High volume boat, sits high in water	Lower volume, sits lower in water
Highly unstable craft	Stable craft
Slow turning, steered by rudder	Fast-turning boat (pivots on centre of boat) steered by paddle
Wing shape paddle for maximum efficiency of each stroke and long shaft for leverage	Flat blade with short shaft for control

This is a power-oriented sport that also requires a good degree of endurance. I suppose it's a bit like circuit or interval training in that respect – in fact intervals and circuits are a great way to train for white water paddling. Learning to use the river and its currents is crucial too, so while fitness is important, the ability to read the water and to know how your boat is going to react is vital. This only comes with practice and experience.

White water racing: this is done in a craft that is higher volume than a slalom craft but still not as unstable as K1. More power is required than in K1 as races last for several miles. An ability to read the water is important as in slalom. Basically you race down a high-grade river negotiating obstacles but racing against the clock to find the fastest route down a raging torrent. This sometimes forces you onto the toughest sections of the river, which require the most physical effort and skill but result in the fastest time. In the television series *Survival of the Fittest* we had a new take on white water racing as we didn't bother with boats! It was a pretty unique experience, as you might imagine, but my ability to read the water meant I beat the other competitors even though some of them were much better swimmers! (One of them was Robin Brew the Olympic medley swimmer. It must be the only time I've beaten him at swimming. See Robin's training programme on pages 60-61.)

Sea/coastal paddling and expedition paddling: this is the water-based equivalent of hiking and exploring. I love getting out around the rugged Dorset coastline and spending a day out in a sea kayak. The craft are made to be stable yet relatively quick to paddle. They have hatches and bungees to attach your kit (a

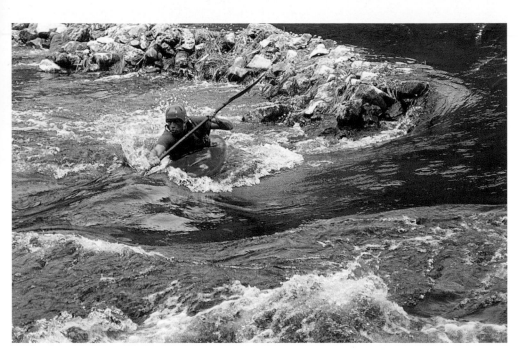

bit like your rucksack for hiking) and often have a built-in compass for navigation.

During my time in the SBS I did my fair share of expedition-type paddling. It was during one of these expeditions that I had my first experience of hallucinations that can occur when you are very fatigued and low on blood sugar! I didn't really believe in the 'pink elephants' that people are always talking about until when paddling past a waterfall on a long selection test, I glanced up and saw a troop of them dancing around in the foam. Needless to say I don't really recommend getting into this state and tend to go for slightly less extreme paddling these days!

If you want to try this great activity, just remember a few basic safety points. You need to let people know where you're intending to go and how long for (just as if you were going hiking). Carry flares and a radio if it's a really serious trip and make sure you know how to use them.

Preferably don't go alone and know the sea states, weather forecast and tides.

The last thing you need is a long paddle against the tide on the way home or to be caught in a serious storm. Finally, use the hatches and storage on the boat to take the necessary food and water and additional clothing. There aren't all that many shops to stop at out at sea!

Canadian canoeing: as well as the kayak, Canadian canoeing is an excellent way of developing teamwork; two guys working a Canadian canoe have incredible harmony, the one at the front providing the power and complementing the captain at the rear. You have the choice of sitting or kneeling as you paddle and it also uses different muscles from kayaking, particularly in the upper and lower back. Canadian canoeing makes a good alternative if you want to try something a bit different on the water. You can simply treat it as a leisure activity and a great way to get into the sport, but you can also race in Canadian canoes.

Symond's Yat: this is where I first experienced the exhilaration of paddling when I was 13. It was a life-changing moment

Rowing

I HAVE ONLY RECENTLY DISCOVERED the pleasures of rowing and ocean rowing and I can't help wishing that I'd been introduced to the sport much earlier; that way I could have experienced more often the fantastic feeling of power you create by transferring the energy of your legs, arms and shoulders into speed across the water.

A couple of years ago I was involved in an attempt to set the world record for rowing between Jersey and Poole. As we were flying out to Jersey, I looked down from the plane and could see Poole harbour in one direction and the Channel Islands in the other. I thought to myself: 'We're going to row all that way?', it was about a hundred miles. We did it and we broke the record – and I was hooked.

Now I regularly go out rowing with a friend in Poole harbour: it's a great buzz, and every so often a couple of the local seals come alongside, just to let us know that we're not alone out there at six o'clock in the morning. This is the time of day for the dedicated pre-work souls: swimmers, kayakers and rowers. There is a satisfying tranquillity, a feeling of contemplative solitude as you push off from the jetty which is soon followed by the euphoria that accompanies hard physical work. You can't help but have a sense of personal achievement, knowing you are out training, relishing the

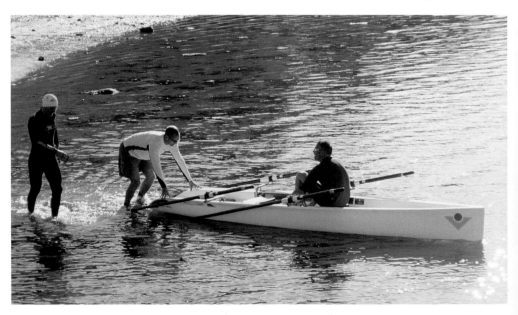

Setting off for a two-hour row. Andy Blow, far left, hopes for a lift

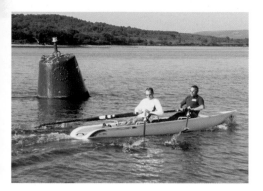

environment while most people are still in bed.

Before I started rowing, I thought that it was just a matter of using your arms, and had no idea about the combination of muscles the sport calls on and the techniques it requires. People often say to me about cycling: 'It looks boring.' I felt exactly the same about rowing and rowing machines until the first time I got in a boat.

As I began to row on a regular basis, I started to see and feel the cross-training benefits: for example, when I run (particularly on a rocky trail) I am aware that I have a lot more strength in my legs and my back. And the same benefits apply to my cycling; again my legs are more powerful.

Although you will gain power from rowing, it is not just a sport for the big guys. The British men's four at the Sydney Olympics included Tim Foster, who was not nearly as big as Redgrave, Pinsent and Cracknell, but he was the master technician who was able to help focus all the power available into making the boat move as efficiently and, consequently, as fast as it did.

The essence of rowing is the explosion of the legs, back and arms as you push back off the footplates, transferring all the power through the blade into the water, followed by an effortless, graceful recovery. That's the theory, although the effortless grace can get more than a bit rocky when you're in choppy water, or you lose the all-important rhythm that is key to good rowing.

I know not everyone has the chance to nip down to Poole harbour for a spot of early morning rowing, but you might be surprised if you check out your local rowing facilities; there are many clubs based on rivers and artificial lakes who will look after you.

If you are not able to join a club or it isn't convenient to do so, then you can use a rowing machine in the gym – or at home. In my opinion a Concept 2 Indoor Rower is just about the only piece of kit you need for your home gym, and if you are rowing on the water as well, it's obviously a superb complementary activity. If you are taught properly how to use the rowing machine and how to plan your rowing programme (see pages 70–71), then you won't be bored. The only problem is you won't get to enjoy the seals!!

Don't be like me and miss out on rowing – I can't recommend it highly enough as a sport for total body conditioning. One old character I know used to go to Ireland 'in his younger days', as he calls them (he was 60 then, so don't ask me how old he is now!) – and row across the whole country from west to east using canals and rivers. Rowing, like cycling, is a sport for life.

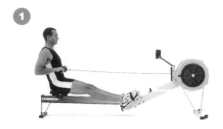

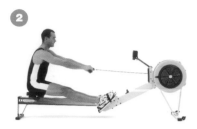

1. The finish: obviously the best place to start! You should be leaning back slightly (think 11 o'clock), with the handle drawn into your belly button, a nice loose grip on the handle, and your forearms horizontal.

2. Here the arms are extended until they are straight and you tilt forwards at the hips while keeping your legs straight. Think 1 o'clock for the body position.

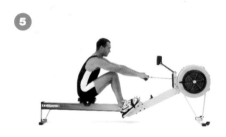

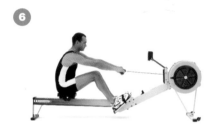

5. As the drive starts you should be pushing away with your legs and subtly levering your torso backwards. Don't simply shove your backside away from the handle with your legs – the whole body needs to work as a unit in this phase, otherwise you won't apply any force to the flywheel.

6. As the drive progresses, the body continues to lever backwards as the legs extend and the arms remain straight. This means that most of the work is being done by the powerful leg, hip and back muscles – not the arms and shoulders as most people think.

The Concept 2 Indoor Rower is not only the market-leading rowing machine but it is also the only piece of fitness kit that has spawned an entire sport and very active following thanks to its accuracy and reliability. Most countries now have a national championship. The British Indoor Rowing Championship is held every year at the National Indoor Arena in Birmingham in November, and there is a British team at the European Championship and the World Indoor Rowing Championship held every February in Boston, USA.

The Concept 2 website has a comprehensive list of Indoor Rowing races in the UK and Europe as well as a very useful training section which includes an interactive training programme developed

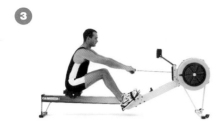

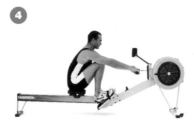

3. The slide: one of the most common errors is to start this phase too early. Make sure that you have completed stage 2 before bending the knees and sliding the seat forwards. You should not have to lift the handle over your knees during the slide phase

4. The drive: at the completion of the slide the seat should not be pressed right up against your heels. This puts your quads in a weaker position for the drive. It is much better to start the drive with your shins vertical.

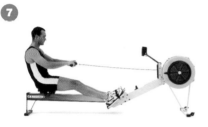

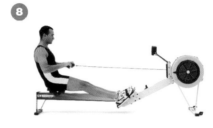

7. As the legs become fully extended and the body finishes leaning back (11 o'clock again), the arms come into play. Avoid the temptation to start pulling with the arms too early as they will tire very quickly.

8. As the arms draw the handle into the body (at belly button height), the torso remains at 11 o'clock, and you are back at the finish position (photo 1 above) ready to start the next stroke. Now get on with it.

by Olympic rowing coach Terry O'Neill. The website also has the Concept 2 rankings which allow you to check out what other people in your country and worldwide are able to do on the Indoor Rower. Becoming a member of the ranking also allows you to keep an online training log and monitor your improvement. The website can be found at www.concept2.co.uk

These pages explain in detail the technique of rowing on a Concept 2 Indoor Rower. It's worth having a good look at them and taking your time to get proficient so that you gain the most from your training sessions. I know that Bernie always cringes when he walks into a health club and sees people hauling away on a Concept Rower with little or no regard for technique. Don't join the purple-faced club, pay attention to what the man says and do it properly! *James Cracknell*

The Concept 2 Indoor Rower

James Cracknell

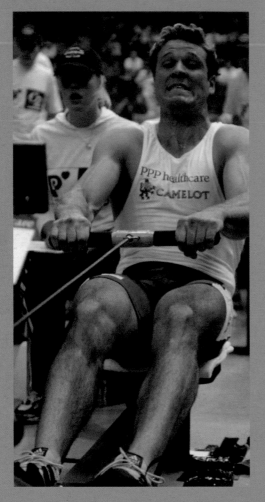

The first thing to say is that it's the best piece of training equipment on land and in my opinion, the most effective. I know it's our rowing action but compared with cycling or skiing inside or outside, the rowing machine is the most efficient workout in terms of total body involvement which you can see from how tired you can get in just a few minutes – so it's a fantastic bit of kit.

Comparing it with being on the water I'd say it has 70–80% similar movement. There are differences: we have a saying about 'ergo minutes' – a minute on the ergo (another name for the indoor rowing machine) is equivalent to two minutes in the boat. On a rowing machine you don't get any of the feelings you get in a boat because when you are in a boat you have the drive phase and the recovery phase, and when you are recovering, the boat is moving under you as it flows over the top of the water.

A lot of our training in the boat is endurance training which means you have time to enjoy the whole environment moving past you. Sitting in a boat that is as wide as the seat on a rowing machine means that you have to balance it – so you've got a lot of different skills to incorporate and you have to be totally in tune with what is going on around you.

Technically it's a lot harder and therefore time passes more quickly. And particularly when you are rowing with a crew, when you are absolutely rowing in time with someone else, when you get it right it's a very sweet feeling. No matter how much you train on the indoor rower you can't replicate that feeling. When you race in a boat, to get as tired in a boat as the rowing machine, you would have to row incredibly well because it's all about timing it with the water. The idea of rowing really efficiently and well is that you can apply more power, so the better you row the more power you can apply and the faster you will go, whereas on the rowing machine you can get away with a bit of poor technique to a certain degree. That's why the top indoor rowers aren't necessarily the best water rowers.

We do use the rowing machine for posture and technique (we always have mirrors in front of the machines). It's used when conditions outside are too windy and also for all our land testing as the machines are so comparable worldwide. See the Concept 2 website for more on how to get yourself a ranking (address on page 71).

We set the machine at level 4 which is the most like rowing on water. In gyms you always see people slam it on level 10, but that's not like rowing, that's more like weight training. Then we do a 2000m or a 5000m test against the clock.

We also regularly do a 30-minute test during which we row as hard as we can, working on power per stroke at only 18 strokes per minute – in fact this is what our whole programme is based on: if you go at a known pace at 18spm you will have a good idea how fast you will go at race pace.

The Concept 2 Indoor Rower is an amazing bit of kit and a massive part of our training. Of course psychologically it is very hard because you get a readout for every stroke, whereas in the boat you get feedback from someone racing next to you or you have to concentrate on being in time, but it's not the same as knowing for a fact you are going this fast (or slow) or that the last stroke was a bit weaker, you're blowing up, you're getting tired, you're getting weak...

The Concept 2 Indoor Rower can really take it out of you, but we couldn't train as effectively without it.

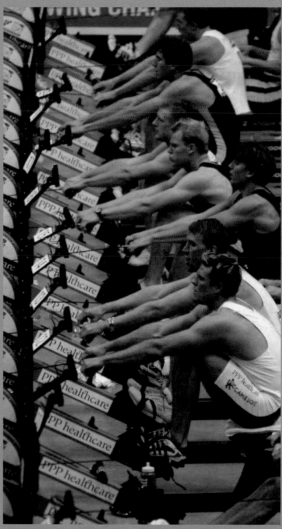

Cross-country skiing

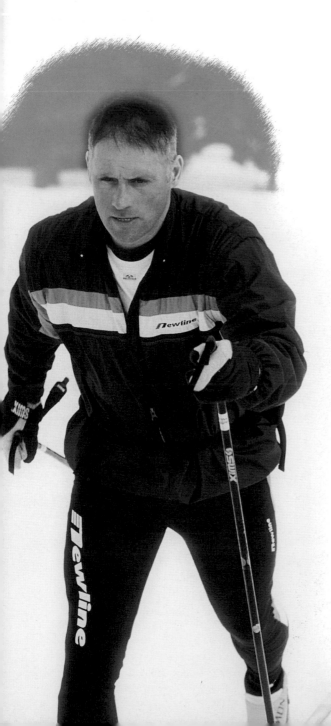

CROSS-COUNTRY SKIING WAS THE FIRST sport that I trained for at any serious level and I quickly discovered (and still believe today) that it is the ultimate sport; it is both demanding physically and is practised in the most stunning environments. When I had the chance to ski in Norway, from the early morning, with the snow crystals glinting in the sun, through to the purple light of the aurora borealis in the evening, the surroundings were breathtaking.

My route into cross-country skiing was as a Green Beret; I applied for 45 Commando, which specialised in mountain and arctic warfare. The mountain training took place on the Isle of Skye, and the arctic training was inside the Arctic Circle in Norway. The basic training included a certain amount of cross-country skiing with sledges and backpacks. I wasn't so keen on digging trenches and sitting in them at –25°C, but the skiing and the wildlife I saw were a revelation – and a genuine inspiration.

The training was demanding: we were doing six to eight hours a day over a ten-day cycle. But I was struck by how graceful the gliding motion was, and started to concentrate on how to master this technique. Neil Bowman, who was in charge of the team, spotted my passion for the sport and my enthusiasm for competition, and thought I might be a good candidate for

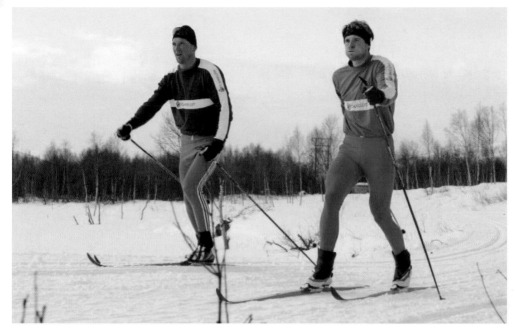

the team he ran.

I'd joined the Marines as a junior. By 1980 I was the British Nordic ski champion in the blue riband event of 15 kilometres. As a kid, that kind of experience was almost unimaginable. Who would have thought that Bernie Shrosbree from Rainham would become the number one Nordic skier in Britain?

When I go to resorts like St Moritz, I see people well into their 70s and 80s still skiing along the ski trails, off to stay in a mountain hut overnight and skiing back into the resort the next day – proof positive that cross-country skiing is one of those sports that you can enjoy throughout your life.

Downhill skiing is, of course, one of Europe's biggest leisure activities. But what horrifies me is that although skiing is a very technical sport, people who only

ski once or twice a year seem to spend most of their preparation time worrying about their salopettes, their accommodation and checking the snow forecasts obsessively – while forgetting to do any more than take the odd lesson.

If you are thinking about going skiing you should really be starting to work on your basic conditioning by the end of the summer. Poor conditioning means poor balance, and you can guarantee that the end result will be serious knee and leg injuries. You can always spot the Brit – he's the one in the Union Jack hat and the plaster cast.

Take away the snow and you begin to understand the problems of skiing without the proper preparations. It would be like racing down Scafell Pike with no training and no balance while relying on two skis.

Cracknell and Pinsent in Norway. One of the many training sessions that day

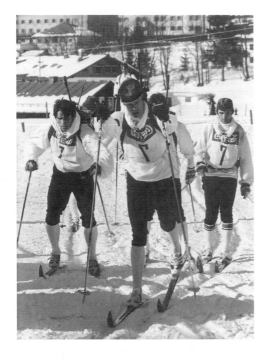

It's hardly surprising that a whole host of groin, shoulder, wrist and elbow sprains are going to happen.

Keeping good balance in whatever conditions you find on the slopes is critical. A fall at any time can be serious, and you need to be resilient. The message is: make sure your body is in good shape for this very demanding sport.

A good training programme to get you ready to hit the slopes would include plenty of core stability training (see pages 104–113), agility exercises such as the hexagon jumps (page 200) and some long, steady aerobic training (jogging, cycling etc.) to give you the stamina to get the most out of those expensive lift passes. It's also a good idea to start 6–8 weeks before your skiing trip; a quick blast in the last seven days is a bit late and won't really help.

If it is the first time that you have been skiing, I recommend that when you get to the resort you spend a couple of days cross-country skiing to help you feel comfortable moving with skis attached to your feet. This also gives you an opportunity to get out and see the forest trails and the beauty they have to offer in a way you can't appreciate when you're pelting down one of the busy slopes.

Benefits of cross-country skiing

As I've already said, I would rate cross-country skiing as the ultimate sport for the fitness gains you can achieve. It combines balance and coordination, power and strength with fantastic aerobic conditioning and is practised in the most uplifting environment in the world.

There's nothing in my mind to beat gliding in freshly cut tracks through snow-clad semi-mountainous Scandinavian locations, working your whole body and knowing there's a hot toddy back at the lodge.

Often cross-country ski trails are at altitude so the aerobic training benefits are enhanced, and using the ski poles on flat and uphill sections develops great upper body strength. Look at pages 106-107 where I tell you how important it is to develop your core conditioning using Swiss balls – now imagine being out on a virgin cross-country ski trail, which, as you learn to balance on the skis, delivers exactly the same core conditioning benefits.

Techniques of cross-country skiing

There are two types of cross-country technique:

• Classic – where ski tracks are already cut into the snow and which you follow like a train. Here you kick the ski through with power and then glide, using the sticks to balance yourself. This is the technique for anyone who enjoys hiking and hill walking. You can take a backpack, ski for three to four hours, stop for a drink at a hut along the way or out in the sun.

• Freestyle – where you employ a skating technique to move over the top of the snow. This was a development of the sport in the mid-1980s, and demands a lot more upper body strength.

You will usually be skiing at altitude. This is going to give your cardiovascular system a pretty good workout, so you need to make sure that you have been working on your aerobic conditioning. It puts demands on your quads, your glutes, the whole hip area, your lower back and shoulders – pretty well all over. You need to train carefully.

During the pre-season I find the best way to train is using rollerskis on tarmac; these are like elongated rollerskates with sticks. The Nordic track machine in your gym will not give you the same feeling. The only machine that gets (even vaguely) close is an elliptical stepper using the ski stick action. As well as training specifically for the skiing action, you can also use crossover training with running and cycling – so either do those activities out of doors or mix in some work on the stepper, bike and treadmill in the gym.

Surprisingly, perhaps, I also suggest you do a lot of rowing. Your immediate reaction might well be that there is little connection

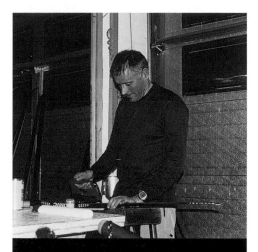

By the way, the thing most people don't realise about cross-country skiing is that you don't just hire or buy the skis and get out there. Preparation of skis is one of the most important issues in the classic style of cross-country skiing. A race can be won or lost on the quality of waxing as the grip for the kick-off to glide or to go uphill is under the foot where the ski is bowed, which is different to the gliding wax on the front and back portions. The type and amount of wax, and how it is applied, depends on the snow temperature, the air temperature and the snow conditions (whether it is old or new snow). It is half science and half an art – top waxers earn nearly as much as the top racers.

between the two sports, but remember that I talked about the amount of upper body strength that cross-county skiing

Waxing: a very special art that makes the difference between winning and losing

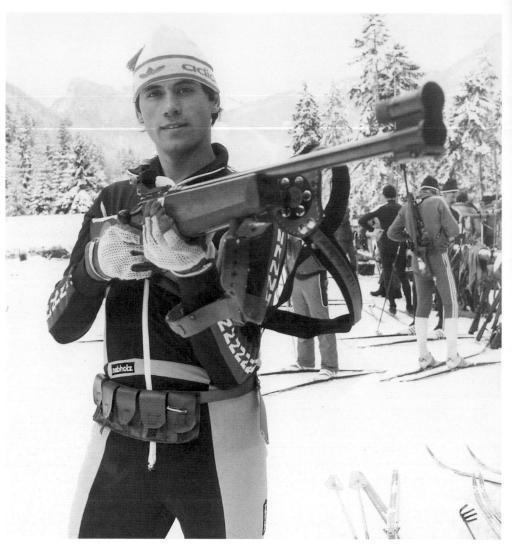

requires. Rowing gives you a workout for the shoulders and back, as well as developing power in the legs. The two sports complement each other perfectly; with the Great Britain Rowing Team we have been using cross-training the other way round for exactly the same reasons.

Rollerblading

This is a great sport, perfect for cities, or flat areas (the Netherlands particularly) and promenades. Like cross-country skiing it is a graceful sport. It has the advantage that it puts less pressure on your knees than running – especially if you're running on pavements or roadways – so you can cover more terrain.

Because your position when rollerblading is that of slightly leaning forward, you need to work on your lower back as well as your core stability. Rollerblading is excellent for improving your cardiovascular capacity, particularly as you can easily control the level of intensity at which you perform.

Ice skating

In the UK we are not blessed with the 60-mile canals that exist in the Netherlands, so opportunities to enjoy this sport are somewhat limited. It's very hard to practise in your local ice rink where the emphasis is on leisure skating, not training.

X-country ski machines in the gym

When these pieces of equipment first started appearing in gyms I have to be honest and say that I was not entirely convinced by their manufacturers' claims that the mechanics were designed to mimic cross-country skiing. I studied them and thought their range of movement was a bit limited and that all of the great aspects of cross-country skiing (balance, core strength and coordination) were missing. However, nowadays I do use them with F1 drivers as a complementary training tool and as a good warm-up and cool down activity, because they are low impact, low resistance and rhythmical to use. For this reason, they're also great for heavier people and those of you getting back into a bit of cardiovascular training after a layoff.

If you're thinking of trying out the wonderful sport that is cross-country skiing and have access to one of these machines, I would recommend some steady state sessions to build up basic fitness. Don't kid yourself that this alone will get you ready for the ski trails though – you'll also need some serious core stability and balance work. Otherwise you might be in for a shock when you hit the white stuff.

Using the cross-training machine

Keep the resistance fairly light so that you can move at a reasonable rate without straining. A reasonable pace is to tap along at 75–85rpm at a Level 3 on the Shrosbree Perceived Exertion Scale (see page 241), i.e. a level of exertion that you would describe as slightly breathless, but able to hold a short conversation.
Increasing the resistance while maintaining the pace will mean that you have to work harder. Unlike the treadmill or exercise bike you may not realise how hard you are working, as the movement is quite unnatural, so keep an eye on your heart rate if you are using a heart rate monitor. This machine is best used for basic conditioning (see pages 90–103).

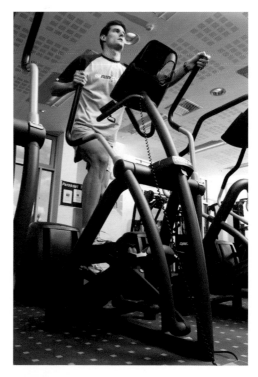

Even Mark Webber is forced to train inside sometimes

Where are you now?

And where do you want to be?

ONE OF THE MESSAGES I WANT TO get across in *Inspired* is that however much encouragement and advice I can give you – and I'll give you as much as I can – ultimately the impetus to get fitter, to improve your performance or to achieve a particular goal, is down to one person. And that person is you.

When you start to notice an improvement in your performance, you will begin to feel very good about yourself. Of course, other people will then also begin to notice and appreciate that your performance is improving (and there's no question that will give you a good buzz), but your true motivation should be to satisfy, and ideally surpass, your own expectations. This in turn will improve your self-esteem, your self-confidence and self-discipline – and then you're ready to take on another set of challenges.

All of that sounds good, doesn't it? But before we start breaking out the bubbly and patting ourselves on the back, you need to decide what it is you personally want to achieve. You might want to compete in a local half marathon. Perhaps you've been on thirty fags a day since you were 20 and want to stop smoking so you can get active and feel healthier in your day-to-day life. Or maybe your sports performance needs to improve by a notch or two to make you more effective in competition.

But even before you start thinking about setting those kind of goals, you have to take a good, honest look at where you are right now.

This is one of the hardest things to do, because we all tend to be in a state of some denial about the true level of our fitness. It's only natural. If you've been stuck behind a desk for the last few years and not doing much, if any, exercise, you will probably have an image in your head of the teenage you, blessed with boundless energy. But is that actually still true? Alternatively, if you're a club athlete, and for some reason your times don't seem to have been improving for a while, you may come up with a whole bunch of external reasons to explain why your performance has plateaued out.

Instead of wasting your energies coming up with a string of excuses, use all that brain time to analyse your fitness in an honest and realistic way. Not only will this give you a baseline to show how you will, quite quickly, begin to see improvements, but it will also get you moving – because it is important to overcome the inertia that lets us think, 'Oh, I'll get round to doing some more exercise soon' and suddenly it's another New Year's Eve and twelve months have slipped by once again.

It's the ultimate dream to have someone with expertise and experience look at you in your current condition and help you to produce a plan of attack to achieve your goals. Whenever I am starting to work with a new athlete, driver or client I spend a lot of time around them while we do some training (and for the really top guys some scientific lab testing). This gives me a chance to suss them out. Are they on time or always late? Are they alert or a bit dopey? What is the level of their technical ability, their motivation to push themselves, their keenness to learn and their ability to act on advice and coaching?

All the time I am watching them train I will be absorbing all this information, and more, to form an educated view of where they are at, how far I believe they can go, and what kind of approach is required.

I realise that not everybody can enjoy – if that's the right word – this level of scrutiny to help them find out where they're at, but I hope it will get across to you the fact that I am not simply interested in how quickly they can run a mile or what their VO2 max is. Where you are at is a state of mind as well as a state of body.

When you come to assess yourself, do not feel nervous about it. You should regard this exercise as a positive challenge – and one that will bring you immediate benefits. A short session of self-assessment helps move you on from the vision you have in your head of the super-fit athlete you would like to be towards the reality of doing something about it.

Right, time for action. Grab a pen and paper for this next bit. Here is your starting point: simply jot down a list of notes about yourself and your body, for example:

- **Do you think you're overweight?**

- **Is your blood pressure on the high side? (Ask your GP for a check)**

- **Do you smoke – and if so, do you want to stop?**

- **How much do you drink a week – do you want to cut back on that?**

- **How much exercise are you currently doing per week? (Be honest – keep a diary of the reality)**

- **What type of aims have you got?**

- **Be realistic – how much time will you genuinely be able to channel into these new activities?**

- **And the big one – how much do you really want it?**

**Be realistic. If you're a month
don't ask me to give you a six-pack
If that's what you want,**

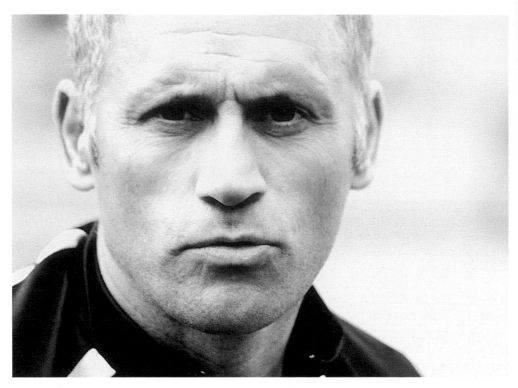

Those of you who are already training regularly, and maybe competing at club level, might also want to add a race or time trial to this list to give you a really good idea of your fitness level. This can compare to your best ever and also to where you have your sights set. It makes a statement of the amount of work that needs doing and means that you can't hide behind the old 'Well, I reckon I'm in shape to do, whatever ...', which is what a lot of people do. Don't reckon – you should really know.

It's also not a bad idea to ask your GP to give you a checkover if you've been out of the loop for a while. He or she will be able to give you an informed and unbiased view of your state of health. Many health clubs will give you a full fitness check too, but remember this is not a substitute for proper medical advice, and you should be a bit sceptical about reading too much into any results you are given.

Have you completed that list now?

Probably the one item in the list that all of us will have ticked is 'weight'. This is a natural side effect of the way we tend to live, that thing of going to the supermarket and thinking, 'The only parking space is four rows back. I can't believe I'll have to walk all that way.' I know, I've done it too. We have all given ourselves far too many comfort zones, and they can easily become addictive. So it's not surprising

away from your wedding,
by the time you go up the aisle.
I've got a chainsaw out the back.

that recent reports have been alerting us all to the fact that, on average, our body shapes are changing and obesity is becoming increasingly prevalent.

I enjoy my quality of life, and that includes good food, good wine and socialising with my friends. I think many people have a vision that I must be some obsessive fitness freak who nibbles on a muesli bar in between 10km runs and 90km bike rides. It's not true – but what I do is make sure that I do plenty of exercise to burn off the food I eat and the odd bottle of red that I enjoy, and I especially try to avoid eating too late in the evening. This just leaves you sleeping overnight with a lot of food swilling around in your gut and very few calories being burnt, which is a great way to become overweight.

If weight is high on your list of priorities, my honest advice is to concentrate on your fitness. The weight loss will follow. You don't need to tie yourself up in difficult and impractical diets; just be sensible and think about moderation. Once you begin exercising in a regular and motivating way, the weight will start to disappear, and that will make you look and feel better. When you've been at it for some time and exercise has become a part of your lifestyle, an upward spiral towards your goals will replace the downward one you might have been experiencing for a while. Don't be unrealistic in your weight loss aims. Losing a few pounds a month is plenty and those pounds will more than likely stay off than if you crash down in ten days by eating like a rodent (despite what all those celebrity-led diets would have you believe).

Goal setting: goals are things you don't need to write down. Matthew Pinsent and James Cracknell don't have to write down in their diaries, 'The goal for this year is to become World Champions again'! They aren't going to forget that. Aims are somewhat different, since those are the stepping stones to achieving a goal. But without an overall goal you are lacking the deep down, vital drive that gets your arse out of the door on a wet cold day. It does not have to be a competitive goal, but it should be something that doesn't come too easily to you – in other words, something you will have to work for. Goals are very individual and wide-ranging, so you need to discover what is inspirational for you.

Writing down aims and goals can create unnecessary pressure and a feeling that missed sessions or events are 'failures', when that is not the case. Becoming unduly fixated with aims and goals is one reason why many people give up training in the early stages – 'I'm not getting anywhere, so I can't be bothered with it anymore.' There is no reason to feel this if you are more flexible with your aims and goals and avoid letting individual blips or the odd bad day distort the bigger picture.

The next stage is to pick a day to make a start. Don't say, 'I'll leave it till the New Year.' Forget the New Year. Start tomorrow. The sooner you begin, the sooner you'll see a change in your body and your performance levels.

At the same time take a look at the shape of your day-to-day life. How many parts of your week are fixed; which are moveable? Can you find a couple of regular slots in the week when you can get out and do some exercising? Treat it like you would a key meeting and schedule in some time. And then give yourself that starting point.

Next, take one simple fixed element: walking round the park or swimming six lengths. Something that is easy for you to monitor on a regular basis. Take a reading of your current time, without pushing yourself to exhaustion – and also, if you can, use a heart monitor and note down the reading from that (for an example, see the heart rate monitor tests on page 87). Remember that this book is all about building up the intensity gradually. Whatever you do, don't start off by deciding that your personal yardstick will be a mile run and rushing off to pound round the local streets with a lot of extra weight bearing down on your out-of-condition joints if you haven't run for a few years, or even months. All this will do is to give you a knee problem that wipes you out for the next six months, and it's back to square one.

If you're starting off after a break from exercise, the best option is probably a brisk walk. As you start working on different aspects of your body, you'll find that the yardsticks of time and heart rate on this walk will naturally improve.

For you club athletes, this is where your race or time trial comes in if you are wanting to get competitive in your sport. Pick a low-key event or a measured route and go for it in a controlled manner – you should not be afraid of the reality of your performance level, even if it's lower

than you want. The information you gain from this is the first step to where you want to be. Armed with your baseline information, you need to start a process of identifying which areas need the most work to improve your performance.

Then set to work chipping away slowly at these factors. Slowly is the key. Don't expect miracles and don't be disheartened if progress is slow. The bottom line is that if you improve steadily for twelve months the improvements you make are likely to be more significant and longer lived than if you blitz things for six weeks, get totally rundown and end up losing the plot.

Allow yourself twelve weeks to build up your general conditioning. Even if you consider yourself pretty active already, it's still good to take three months to build up all-round, total body conditioning. It may take three to four weeks for your creaking joints, dodgy tendons and that back that's been playing up to start remembering how they are designed to work. The classic principle of 'Longer, Lower, Regular' should be your mantra in this phase!

At this point you've acquired a certain amount of data about your physical condition, and you've started thinking about yourself in a straightforward and honest way. Above all, you're already doing something. And not just talking about it. We're under way.

Fitness is a very personal thing. There are a number of different ways of measuring the performance of your body, but I actually think the true definition of fitness is qualitative rather than quantitative. It's about finding your own form.

There is an American definition which

Take your time. And make sure you master the basics first. You wouldn't dream of building a house without laying the foundations first.

runs, 'Fitness is the ability to carry out a given task to meet your daily needs.'

That phrase carries a great meaning for me because it gets across that fitness means different things to different people. For a sprint swimmer like Mark Foster 'fit' means being in fantastic condition to be able to swim 50m flat out in 21 seconds: he probably wouldn't be fit enough to compete with the best in the world over 1500m – an event which lasts for 14 or 15 minutes, although he would be far fitter than most office workers. Equally, a bricklayer who carries hods up and down ladders all day would be lapped endlessly in a track race against Haile Gabrselassie, but I reckon it would be Haile who would be hanging out his backside if he had to shift a dozen breeze-blocks up three flights of stairs! Which of them is the 'fittest'? A lot of it depends on the task you are talking about. What you need to do is think about what fitness means to you.

There is nothing more discouraging than allowing yourself to set over-optimistic, if not downright delusory, goals. It is no good declaring that your goal is running a four-minute mile if you can't yet run a ten-minute mile. You may be going out and training hard but you will lack that vital sense of achievement. Sometimes this can lead to people training harder and harder simply because they are not achieving the excessively high goals they set themselves; they are working themselves to death in the gym and still feeling unsatisfied and unhappy.

Don't be impatient. And never over-train. Remember that at the highest level of sports, athletes increase their training level very, very gradually.

You should be aiming to finish every session thinking to yourself, 'That was a great session.' It is very easy to push yourself to exhaustion. The difficult – but most rewarding – thing is to find the right balance between what enhances you both physiologically and psychologically. Your body and your mind should feel lifted by the session – if you can achieve that, you've won the main battle.

Don't over-analyse yourself.
It can quickly become another excuse for never actually doing anything. My message, when I can see that somebody is spending too long agonising over a problem or worrying about the next challenge is simply, 'Shut up, and make it happen.' That sounds brutal, but it's true. I was teaching a group of people to abseil. There was one girl who had come along to watch her friends, and she kept talking about how she would never be able to abseil. In the end, she was so wound up about it, she had to have a go, even though – in her head – she hated the idea. She went over the edge of the cliff, and loved it. I could see the fire in her eyes when she finished the abseil, and the pleasure and self-belief she had gained from confronting and dealing with her fear.

Heart rate monitors

And a basic fitness test

THE HEART IS, WITHOUT DOUBT, THE most important muscle in the body. Fortunately it is one of the easiest muscles to train and that can have a big impact on your overall health. Although the workings of the heart are very complicated, your heart rate (or HR for short) pulls together a whole range of physiological factors and is described in one very simple figure: beats per minute (e.g. 130bpm).

At rest, average heart rate values vary between 60 and 80bpm and this figure can be used as an indicator of improving health, fitness and performance. When you become fitter your heart becomes stronger, and your resting heart rate can decrease as the heart has the improved ability to pump more oxygenated blood around your body when required. During exercise, heart rates can, in some people, exceed 200bpm – depending on fitness levels, age and other factors. There are a number of reasons why an individual's heart rate will vary and will also differ from another person's; these include stress, ambient temperature, medication, fitness levels, genetics and even the position that you are sitting in right now! There is even a difference in heart rates between men and women for the simple reason that women tend to have slightly smaller hearts and they, therefore, need to work a little harder to maintain the same level of intensity during strenuous activity. I often come across club athletes chatting in the changing room about just how high they have managed to get their heart rate during a training session or race. They seem to be very impressed with high numbers, but don't always seem to understand what the term heart rate means; you, on the other hand, will have, by now, already started to appreciate that your heart rate is completely individual to you.

So why do we need to measure heart rate if it is in continual use 24 hours a day, 7 days a week, 52 weeks of the year? From an exercise point of view, the answer is quite simple – your heart rate is a fairly reliable indicator of how hard you are training and if you train too hard then you can become injured. You may 'overtrain' which in some instances can be dangerous. If you do not train hard enough then you will not achieve your fitness and training goals and will waste time! Therefore by using a heart rate monitor (such as the Polar models shown here) you can accurately monitor training intensity and take the guesswork out of exercise. And what is more important is that you will achieve your training goals in a shorter time – by training at the right intensity for the required amount of time.

For example, in endurance sports the important factor is not the out-and-out high level of the heart rate you achieve, but the ability to work at a very high percentage of your personal maximum heart rate. A club athlete who has a personal maximum of 190bpm and who can sustain a rate of 175bpm in a race (i.e. working at 92% of their maximum heart rate) could well be beaten by a top performer who only runs at 170bpm, but has a max of 175bpm, and so is working at a much higher percentage of his or her maximum heart rate.

Heart rate training has been studied in academic institutions for many years and is a complex subject, but you don't need a sports science degree to appreciate and apply the basics of the subject to your training. For a long time I have been using a chart of 'perceived exertion' along with heart rate monitor information to simplify the explanation of training intensities and to relate them to individual athletes across a wide range of sports. Using a heart rate monitor and the Shrosbree Perceived Exertion Scale (SPES) on page 241, you can note down your personal heart rates against the six different levels on the chart and this will help you train using a combination of science and 'feel factor'.

A basic fitness test for everyone

I've outlined here a basic fitness test that provides the essential elements of heart rate monitoring protocol; it will give you an easy to apply, albeit rough and ready, idea of your basic aerobic fitness. Find a route to walk around that is fairly flat, will give you 15–25 minutes of walking time and is, importantly, interruption free (i.e. with no road crossings involved). Put your heart rate monitor on and walk at a brisk pace that you will be able to sustain for the full distance. Make a note of your time at a couple of points along the way to help with your pace judgement the next time you repeat the session. You should get quite warm walking at this pace, so don't overdress and overheat as this will simply

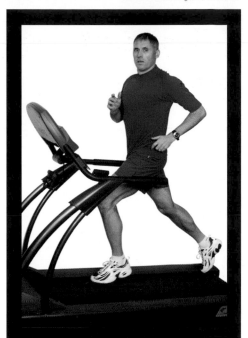

Here's an interesting question. Why does your heart rate get higher and higher if you run on the treadmill at a constant speed in the gym for 20 minutes or more? The answer is a phenomenon which is known as 'cardiovascular drift'. When you start exercising, particularly in a warm environment, your body temperature rises and you begin to sweat. The water in your sweat has to come from somewhere and a certain proportion is drawn from the plasma in your blood. This has the effect that the total volume of blood in your body starts to decrease. Therefore, to maintain good blood flow to the muscles which are working, the heart has to work that little bit harder to sustain the same level of activity, and as a result your heart rate increases. Incidentally, this is part of the reason why taking on fluids is important during exercise and obviously the effect of cardiovascular drift is magnified in any hot and humid conditions.

push up your heart rate. Make a note of the time it takes you to complete the route, your average and maximum heart rates for the session and, if possible, download the data from your heart rate monitor onto your computer via the infra-red interface – this will give you a graph of your heart rate over the time it took to complete the walk.

After 4–6 weeks of training go back and repeat the session. Walk at exactly the same pace (this is where the split times to certain staging points will help) and again record your time and your average and maximum heart rates. If you can, download this onto the computer to overlay the graph from the previous trial. You should find that your average and maximum heart rates are lower for the second trial. You will also probably have found that it felt easier to complete the exercise at the same pace. If not, it may be time to review the training you have been doing (or not doing) and to check that no other factors have affected your performance.

For each test you should monitor those factors that are under your control and try to keep them the same. That means picking days with similar temperatures, wearing the same clothing and doing the tests at the same time of day. Don't bother undertaking the test if you are feeling unwell or tired, or if you have been rushing about like crazy. Trying to squeeze

the test in between stressful events in your life will only give you a distorted view of where you are currently at.

You should also bear in mind that cigarettes, caffeine in drinks and any prescription medications can affect your heart rate.

I prefer this kind of self-test to going out and working from heart rate zones predicted by the '200 minus your age' formula, which is often wildly inaccurate. The basic fitness test tells you what your heart rate will be at Level 3 on the SPES and just what it feels like. As you get fitter you can go out and work harder to establish your heart rate zones for exertion Levels 4, 5 and occasionally 6. What I mean by this is that rather than relying on maths and theories to generate your heart rate training zones, take the time to get to know your body and 'feel' the zones described in the SPES, then match your heart rates to them by keeping an eye on your monitor during training. Periodically, back this up with the basic fitness test to see what progress you are making.

Remember that becoming familiar with your 'zones' may take months and, just to confuse things, your zones and the respective heart rates will shift around as you get fitter, but that is the beauty of the system – it grows (or withers) with you as your fitness changes.

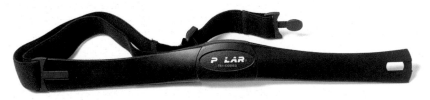

Types of heart rate monitors

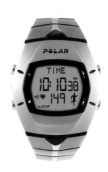

F92ti: equipped with leading-edge training technology and the most sophisticated features a serious health club user would need – Ownzone, Owncal, Owncode, Ownindex Test and a whole lot more – the F92ti is both a stylish and invaluable piece of kit.

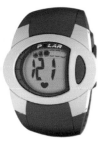

F1: an entry level HRM that provides an accurate heart rate and total exercise time.

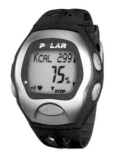

F5: a more sophisticated HRM with a range of additional functions including average heart rate and calorie consumption during the exercise session.

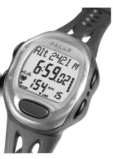

S720i: designed for cyclists with a built-in altimeter and thermometer and a range of specific cycling functions including speed average and maximum, a wireless speed sensor and distance based recovery measurement.

POLAR. www.polar-uk.com

You'll get the most out of your exercise and use your time most efficiently if you're exercising at an effective intensity level. How do you know where you are? Heart rate. It's that simple. Your heart rate is a convenient, reliable indicator of your exercise intensity, and with a heart rate monitor, that indicator is as convenient as a glance at your wrist. They work with a transmitter belt you wear around your chest to detect the electric signal emitted from your heart. The belt then sends an electromagnetic signal to the wrist receiver, which shows you accurate information about your heart rate. Armed with this information, you're well equipped to make decisions about and adjustments to your workout, varying it depending on your fitness level and your goals for exercising.

Basic conditioning

BASIC CONDITIONING IS A PHRASE that is bandied about a lot in sports training, but is frequently misused and usually misunderstood. When I use the term 'basic conditioning', I am talking about creating the starting point for any person at any level of fitness. The same term can apply whether we're talking about someone who has decided that they want to start off virtually from scratch with some exercise in the home or the local gym, or an elite sports performer who has had a layoff because of injury or an end-of-season break and needs to begin their training and exercise over again.

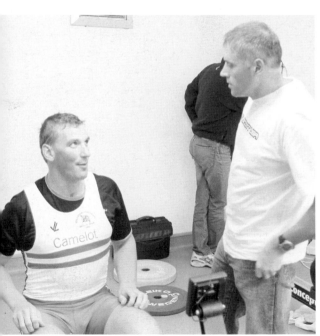

The first key element in good basic conditioning is flexing one vital part of your anatomy – the brain – because good basic conditioning is all about careful analysis of yourself and identifying areas of weakness that you need to enhance. I think of it like taking out an insurance policy, which prevents you from over-committing yourself, or overstraining yourself later on.

Mark Allen, the great Ironman champion, always used to say, 'The successful elite performer is the one who can train the most consistently without getting injured or ill.' That's a quote that gets to the root of why basic conditioning is so important for all of us, and especially anyone who is exercising regularly. For elite performers, it is very, very demanding to go out training three or four times a day without becoming worn down or getting ill. In professional sport this is a problem which has become worse over recent years, as the demands of money and television make it increasingly difficult for top athletes to get a break. In soccer, there was once a time (I'm showing my age) when the main match was on Saturday afternoon, with plenty of time to recover during the following week. Now the schedule demands up to three matches a week. In these circumstances, basic conditioning becomes extremely important.

Do you think you've really earned your sandwich, Matthew?

Right people. Pay attention to this. It's the most important section in this book, so make sure you take it all in.

For non-professionals, the same thing applies. There is no point training for six weeks for an event and then ripping your hamstring. Of course, you can be unlucky – accidents do happen – but if you are planning a skiing holiday or wanting to enjoy a good club season in your own sport, you will find the risks of that kind of injury are drastically reduced if you commit to a basic conditioning programme.

There is one common problem that people encounter when they start this kind of training. Basic conditioning tends to be something that everybody wants to avoid, especially club sportsmen and women. If I'm working with somebody and suggest to them that we concentrate on doing one particular routine or exercise, and then they say, 'Oh, I hate that', it's usually a good sign that here is an area to concentrate on. Start learning not to always do your favourite exercises. If you're following a programme at the gym, and you automatically take out that sweaty bit of dog-eared card for every session, ask yourself when was the last time you really reviewed the overall shape of the programme, rather than just increasing the weights and repetitions? There are so many people doing the same sessions blindly every week, it scares me.

Similarly if you rely on top-of-the-range equipment, it doesn't mean you're the best. All the hi-tech kit in the world won't help you perform out on the road or on the field. At the Henley gym, where the Great Britain Rowing Team train, there are just some basic weights and rowing machines. Or think of those boxing clubs where the apparatus is simple (and the changing rooms usually have some unspecified growths) but the results are self-evident.

I remember a time when I was doing cross-country skiing in 1978; I hated one particular course because it was extremely hilly with a lot of sharp climbs. I was fine on long climbs because I had good basic endurance. But where I was weak was on the short climbs. I went back home and concentrated specifically on some basic conditioning for that aspect of my fitness with a series of sand dune climbs and hill bounding. Two years later I was the British Nordic ski champion. OK – it wasn't quite as simple as that, but I had been able to identify a weakness in my sport and put a programme in place to improve it.

Arthur Lydiard, who coached the legendary New Zealand distance runner Peter Snell, would always give his athletes a base of endurance work over a period of years heading towards their final goal, so that when they came to perform in the Olympic 800 metres final, for example, that one race represented the peak of months and years of carefully planned preparation.

He made a very good point: that this phase of 'basic conditioning' should last as long as possible. In his view if you could spend six months on basic conditioning, so much the better. My personal feeling is that I would always like to see people undertaking 8–12 weeks of general conditioning work. In other words, basic conditioning is not about pitching up for three sessions a week for a fortnight or so and then loading yourself up with the heavy weights. If you do that, it's a gamble. You might get away with things for a while, but more than likely something will crack or snap before too long.

For me, generally speaking. people tend to fall into one of two categories: either they do no basic conditioning at all or they only do conditioning and it becomes their entire way of training, full stop.

Look at it as a preparation for your actual training. Although you will probably see substantial improvements at the beginning of any programme of basic conditioning, that is not what you are really aiming for. Rather than a series of peaks and troughs, you should see a very gradual improvement over a long period of time.

This is a fine art, and that's why good coaches are invaluable for a top performer; they are able to control and manage the minute increases in performance. It's in our nature to look for short cuts in everything, but in the twenty years I've been around the high end of sport, I've yet to find a single short cut

that really works.

For your own basic conditioning programme, the first thing to do is to create a shopping list of the areas you need to work on – cardiovascular, strength, or the whole package. As I said in the last chapter, look at where you are and where you can realistically get to. What have you always had a problem with?

I am sure your body will have told you in a fairly blunt way. If you've been out hiking in the hills for a few days and your back aches so much you can't wait to get into a hot bath each evening, that is a straightforward and difficult-to-ignore message that you have not been conditioning your lower back. Let your body do the talking – and listen to it. That's how you will develop the personal interpretation and control of your own training, rather than just following the same old routine, or relying in a rather lazy way on a personal trainer to write out your programme for you. That's not to say you shouldn't use a good personal trainer; just try to work with them so that you have an input into your own programme – don't just shift the

DOMS stands for 'delayed onset muscle soreness' (i.e. it hurts like hell!) and will arise 24–48 hours after a fairly intensive bout of activity using muscles not normally employed in your usual training. A classic example is the vigorous game of squash you played on Saturday afternoon that leaves you feeling like you've been in the ring with Lennox Lewis when you try to get out of bed on Monday morning. It is a combination of microtears in the muscle and damage caused by the waste products of high intensity activity. The good news is that in and of itself DOMS is not usually a long-term problem, but it's a good indicator that your basic conditioning needs fine tuning before you go out and do again whatever activity caused it.

Remember that conditioning is the point when you identify the things you need to work on. Conditioning is the precursor to training.

responsibility onto someone else entirely. Get involved and the whole process will be more enjoyable and rewarding.

When you start on basic conditioning, keep going. Continuity is vital; it's no good doing five weeks out of eight and then stopping. Every week lost will require two to three weeks to get back on track with your improvement. How many people have bought an exercise bike in the New Year after too much festive cheer, and then only used it half a dozen times? The reason, generally, is that they have failed to understand why they are doing the exercise, and that in turn leads to boredom. There's no understanding, no enjoyment. This is an era in which we have become used to instant gratification, and basic conditioning is absolutely not about that. Always understand why you are doing exercise. Start understanding yourself today. You will need that as well as some commitment. This book could take you twelve months to absorb, but if you stick with it, and me, I know you will start seeing the benefits.

If you spend time focusing and visualising your own goals (and nobody else's, especially not the person at the next machine) I guarantee you will see payback in other areas of your life. The bottom line of this book is there is no easy way; you have to get off your arse and do it...

Now, I know everyone is different, but here are three useful and typical descriptions of people. You can choose (and be brutally honest with yourself!) which of these is nearest to your own attitude and level of fitness, and have a look at the kind of basic conditioning they are doing.

Type 1: Out of condition/no history of fitness training or sport

This is the person known to the rest of the world as a couch potato, and to me as the pie thief ... In this case almost any exercise is better than no exercise. Even so, the basic conditioning must be structured.

A colleague at the Renault F1 Team came to me to get him fit. He won't mind me saying he fell absolutely into this category. First, I asked him to simply walk on the treadmill three times a week, which was actually very hard for him to do as it amounted, in his terms, to 30 minutes of reasonably vigorous exercise. This was gradually increased, in small increments, to five sessions of 45 minutes a week and then we started to introduce some circuit type weights and resistance work. He really started enjoying the improvement he could see and feel; so many people rush out to the gym, and then the initial euphoria fades fifteen minutes later. Here we were able to create a growing sense of achievement that continually renewed his enthusiasm. The actual level of exercise suggested in this situation may be relatively modest, but it represents an easy start – and the progression from nothing to something is amazing.

If you're in this category, your basic conditioning might consist of a walk outdoors three times a week. Or you could walk to the fridge and get your own beers out instead of sending the missus! Funnily enough, I also find that it is this group, 'the pie thieves', who always tell me they are too busy to do any sessions (too busy making excuses, usually).

In order to make a progression, move

from three sessions of 10 minutes in week one, up to 12/13 minutes a session the following week, and so on. Your aim should be to accumulate regular sessions and time spent. It is not about the speed you are going at, but about the volume and extent of the work you can commit to. Once you have reached 30–45 minutes a session that is your first plateau: twelve weeks of that will be an excellent start. You can then start adding gradients or walking with dumbbells to increase the difficulty factor.

Type 2: **Active sports history but out of practice**

I call this type Mr or Ms Normal: it's someone who uses a computer at work every day, and who once did quite a lot of squash or soccer or tennis at a social or semi-competitive level, but has lost the habit. This type of basic conditioning is like taking an old car out of the garage and giving it a good, thorough service.

It pays to start off at a low level and gradually get a feel for where your body is working easily, and where it is having problems, so that you can build up confidence before moving on to the higher intensity work. Unlike the total beginner, you can go straight into some brisk walking and jogging, and undertake exercises in the gym that place a wider range of more technical demands on the body and which provide a level of resistance and dynamic movement: the rowing machines or the free weights for example.

In this category, you should look at doing the heart rate monitor (HRM) fitness test set out on pages 87–88. This will give you a good idea of where you are at and provide a genuine yardstick for future reference.

And if you haven't been in the gym since you picked up your shiny new membership card, make sure you spend a couple of weeks getting to know the individual machines, and acquiring a feel for the environment. Get on the machines and understand the feedback they give you. This is great for motivation but don't start running yourself into the ground on the treadmill, as it will only end in tears. Aim for three or four sessions per week and build up to 60 minutes plus per session. When you have got a good, honest two to three months of this type of training under your belt you can start setting a few challenges and upping the intensity for a couple of sessions a week. This will provide the subtle overload needed to create a bit more form and fitness and take you to the level you really need to get back into your sport.

Type 3: **The club athlete and beyond**

Sometimes the club athlete is a nightmare. He or she always wants to get straight out there and start performing because they are blessed, or cursed, with an excess of enthusiasm. They ignore the basic conditioning, get hurt, and then have to go all the way back to square one. Elite, professional athletes tend to have more structured and personalised training, so they are unlikely to avoid basic conditioning, but even so you can always find areas to work on.

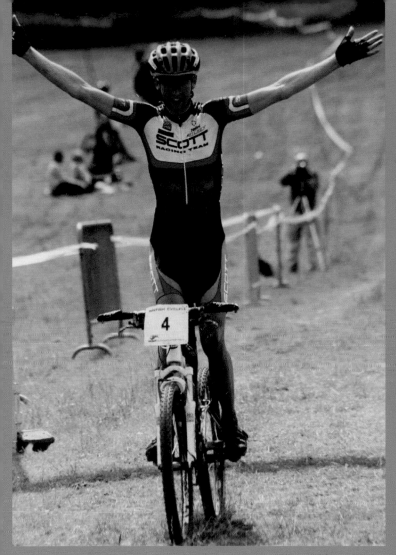

specific condition will never be the best it can be. It made sense to me: despite thinking I had good condition and core strength my assessment proved that I was seriously lacking; I was good for an average person but not for a world-class athlete, which is what I wanted to be.

In the off-season I cross-trained, skipped, swam, rowed, and hammered the core stability. I also did some nasty circuit training. By the time I started working on my bike I was a better athlete and as a result fatigued slower and suffered fewer injuries.

In the following years and when my general condition was good enough I started weight training. Mixing general condition exercises and bike-specific movements led to increased strength, which I could then transfer as more endurance and power on my bike. By looking at things from a general perspective I have gained improvements in my own sport.

Oli Beckingsale

I started to work with Bernie in 2001. I had been a professional mountain biker for three years and in 2000 had competed at the Olympics. Despite some successes I was not really reaching my potential and was not progressing at the rate I would have liked.

I was training in a cyclist way, a bit old school, which involved riding my bike a lot and not much else. I was doing some modern training but it was all cyclist-based and bike-specific.

In our early meetings, we looked at my general condition. Bernie's view is that if the general condition is not there, the

Don't spend all your money on the latest machines or gadgets. Invest in intelligence and experience.

It's hard to generalise for these guys because the basic conditioning is so related to their own sports and disciplines. However, here are a couple of examples to start you thinking about it.

Mountain bike champion Oli Beckingsale came to work with my team in the January of one year. He had started basic conditioning in the previous November, so he was eight weeks into the conditioning phase. We identified that aerobically he was very efficient, but he was missing out on strength in his core region, on explosiveness and speed. He had the honesty to admit that he never moved away from his programme so we changed the mix around, dropping his bike work down to two sessions a week, but bringing him into the gym five times a week. Then we increased the bike work to four sessions a week. At the end his physio said that he had never seen Oli in such good shape.

Andy Blow, who works with me, is a national-level triathlete, with a strong academic background in sports science. When I saw his swim training programme in the conditioning phase – long swims for distance and volume – I simply asked him what was going on in his head: his mind was too fixed on delivering the distance and the times, not on his technique. I got him to swim shorter distances and to concentrate on his technique instead because for some people conditioning is as much about technical efficiency as physical preparation. Also Andy wasn't able to observe himself swimming. As I walked along the poolside watching his swimming motion I copied it, so that I could feel what he was doing. I had a couple of suggestions to help his technique which he tried, saw the benefits of and adopted out of his own choice because he could see genuine results in his performance. I don't have any formal coaching qualifications for swimming, but I have learnt what to feel and what to look for.

What it all comes down to is my version of an academic approach: which is using your mind, but combining that with experience and intuitive understanding of what's needed.

Endurance base work for basic conditioning

I want to take the opportunity here to expand on the subject of basic conditioning for endurance sports. This is an area of massive interest to me as a result of all the years I spent competing, and I also reckon it's an area where loads of athletes today make the mistake of skimping and cutting corners; a fatal mistake if you want to race competitively over a long season.

I learned a lot about basic conditioning for endurance sports from watching cross-country skiers in Scandinavia. The Finns and Norwegians were great at the long-distance races and trained over huge distances during the off season. Neil Bowman, who was my mentor in the sport, taught me that the Nordic approach was to build an incredible endurance base in this way, to provide the underlying strength which allowed them to race week in and week out during a whole season.

He also taught me that whenever you

are doing any endurance work, the way to avoid boredom is to spend your time constantly thinking about and analysing the activity while you're doing it. Keep your brain working at all times. It is the perfect chance to think about the 'souplesse' of your movement when cycling (see page 49). If you're running, concentrate on the rhythm of your movement (see page 33). In both swimming or kayaking, try to improve your feel for the water (see pages 58–59) so that good technique will be deeply embedded in your mind and body for when race day dawns.

To give you an idea of the kind of time that the best endurance athletes spend on endurance base work, I often refer people to the following quote from Lance Armstrong, the legendary Tour de France winner. It was actually said in response to doping allegations falsely made against him: 'I'm on my bike six hours a day busting my ass. What are you on?' I'm sure he wasn't exaggerating either!

I know that some people are not too convinced by the idea of high volume training, particularly for 'shorter' endurance events that only last up to, say, two hours – why do three to five hour sessions when you'll only ever race over half that time? Quality not quantity, they cry, and to a certain extent I agree. In the specific, short-term build-up for events quality sessions at or above race pace are a must with big recovery time to allow for the best performance on the day. However, neglecting the base and quality work will only allow you to get so far and hold your form for a limited time. Base

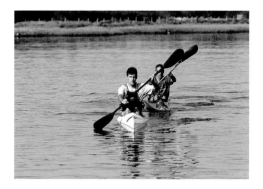

work done at a demanding but sensible pace will give the mental toughness, physical robustness and technical attention to detail that allows you to train harder in quality phases and reach higher, more sustained peaks when they occur. Get fit quickly with a diet of fast intervals and low volume work and sooner or later it will bite you on the backside – I've seen it many times and have also seen the guys and girls who got their basic endurance conditioning right go on to achieve stunning results.

So, that's the theory. The practice for you is to look at your sporting activity and your sporting performance and list your weaknesses: these are the areas where you know you need to concentrate on the Lower, Longer, Regular work. Make yourself a shopping list.

It will work. I trained a local mountain biker who was extremely sceptical about the value of endurance work. At the beginning he couldn't see why we had to do so much low intensity work when what he really wanted to achieve was speed. I explained my reasoning and he stuck with it. Now he's number 2 in his national age group. Say no more...

What do we mean by aerobic and anaerobic training?

THE WORDS 'AEROBIC' AND 'Anaerobic' are commonly heard in the jargon used by fitness instructors and gym-goers – often used inappropriately and out of context I might add!

Basically the terms are used in the world of physical training to describe the processes used by the body to convert stored energy into activity; aerobic means 'with oxygen' and anaerobic means 'without oxygen' and this should give you a clue about how they relate to training.

Unfortunately for some years there has been an over-simplification of the terms to the point where most go-get-fitters seem to believe that when you train at an easy pace it equals aerobic training and then suddenly, as you train harder, the body flicks a switch and 'bang' you are into anaerobic training mode. The reality is that the body is constantly drawing energy from both aerobic and anaerobic sources all of the time – it's just the proportions that vary, with easy to steady activities being predominantly fuelled by aerobic sources (as the oxygen being inhaled is sufficient to meet the demands made in the muscles) and with sprinting, weightlifting or explosive-type activities having to rely on energy that is supplied instantly and produced without oxygen (as the supply can't keep up with the demand).

Anaerobic energy supplies are fine for this short-term activity but do have the downside of producing waste products such as lactic acid and carbon dioxide. It is these toxins, as they build up in the body tissues, which make anaerobic efforts so painful. The same is not true of aerobic supply, which means that if enough fuel and energy are available it is theoretically possible to keep exercising aerobically indefinitely.

It is true that there is a kind of 'threshold' above which the level of anaerobic energy required creates an overwhelming demand on the body and you have to back off to be able to keep going. This has been called the anaerobic threshold, the lactate threshold and all sorts of other names. Basically, the terms refer to the point where you increase from exercising at a

Longer, Lower, Regular is an uncomplicated and memorable way of explaining how to condition for endurance. You do exactly what it says and stay out of the red-zone or high intensity work. I had arrived at this simple mantra after several seasons of training for Nordic ski events, but the importance and power of the phrase really struck home when I first met Professor Clyde Williams at Loughborough University who said, 'Bernie, you have just condensed my 2-hour lecture on endurance training into three words!' So now all his sports science students learn about Longer, Lower, Regular in their first term.

Steady state training will vary from sport to sport and different coaches will use the phrase to describe various training regimes, but essentially it means training at or just below the anaerobic threshold. I usually describe this as training in the 'comfort zone at just below race pace'. It's used for long interval training, e.g. running for 4-8 miles or cycling for 10-25 miles and is all about sustaining the activity for a reasonable amount of time.

steady rate that feels hard but sustainable to a rate that sends your breathing rate through the roof and you quickly realise that you are going to have to slow down or stop very, very soon! This, however, is not the same as simply 'switching' from one supply to another as the process gradually adapts as your pace goes up by providing more and more anaerobic energy until your systems can't cope with the levels of waste products any more. Incidentally, raising this threshold is the Holy Grail for a lot of endurance athletes who want to race as close to it as possible as it represents the optimum level of performance in steady state events.

In terms of what this means in day-to-day training, activities that are classified as 'aerobic' are generally steady, rhythmic exercises like jogging, cycling, rowing, stepping – when they are done at a controlled rate. It is of course possible to train more anaerobically at these activities by pushing the pace up to a high level, but you will only ever manage this sort of intensity for relatively short periods of time as the by-products of anaerobic metabolism build-up in the body tissue.

Certain activities like weightlifting are much more anaerobic in nature as they require a short burst of activity with a rest period immediately after. This rest is necessary for the muscles to be replenished with fuel (mainly something called ATP–PC if you want to impress your mates) and to clear the built-up waste by-products from the tissues. This goes a long way to explain why sprint athletes seem to spend a lot of their training time sitting around between bouts of furious but brief activity. It can take several min-

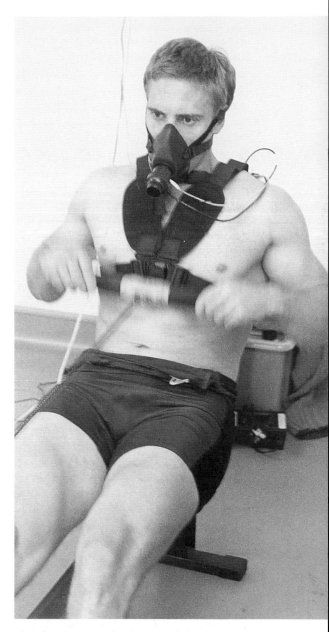

utes for the muscles to completely recover from only 10 seconds of flat-out work before it can be repeated to good effect!

Pete Gardner, a member of the GB Rowing Team, undergoes a VO2 max test

Cardiovascular equipment in the gym

The misuse I see of CV kit in the gym never ceases to amaze me. Few people, it seems, understand either their functions or how to use them properly, especially as part of a training plan. Most treadmills are now quite advanced with shock absorption systems designed to cushion the initial impact of your footstrike and with all sorts of computerised enhancements. These are, in fact, very good machines indeed – when used correctly. It still astounds me though, to see many people running on them in totally inappropriate footwear. You need to wear a pair of proper running shoes as if you were out on the road. Strength training footwear or cross-training shoes won't offer the support and cushioning you need and you are risking injuries.

Once you've got the correct shoes on, I am going to assume that you have more or less gone straight from the changing rooms to the machine. OK, turn it on and start with a brisk walk increasing to a light jog for a few minutes and then get off to do a little bit of mobility work (to loosen up your joints). Now get back on to do your main session. Incidentally, for a gentle walking pace set the machine at around 5kph, for brisk walking you can get up to 7 or 8kph. Whatever you plan to do for the next ten, fifteen or even sixty minutes, you must begin with the warm-up phase otherwise you are risking an injury and you won't get the best out of your session. In addition, most gyms and health clubs position these machines in front of mirrors so you can actually look at your running form, style and mechanics (did you think the mirrors were there so

you could admire your new designer kit?) – so that's what you should use them for.

A poor way to train is to simply power up the machine from cold with the sole intention of busting a gut, worrying about how much you've gained over the last session, how many more miles you are going to cover in a given time or how many Mars bars you will burn off. And don't be misled by the 'calorie counters' on most of these machines; ninety-nine times out of a hundred, the figures they churn out are as accurate as your weekly lottery numbers and about as much use.

Far better is to aim to run continuously for twenty minutes at a steady state pace, feeling quite relaxed, and using your heart rate monitor, watching your heart rate curve – it should just drift up gradually throughout those twenty minutes. You should feel like you have to concentrate on what you're doing, but be able to hold a brief conversation with someone if you needed to.

For someone completely new to these machines, well you just need to get on one and, after the warm-up phase, simply walk briskly, getting used to how the platform or belt feels underfoot. Then progress to jogging and then move on to jogging with efficiency – that is by upping the speed to a comfortable level and keeping it constant thereafter. Eventually you can progress to some small intervals when you go slightly quicker for thirty seconds and then come down to a jog for a minute, then go up reasonably hard again for thirty seconds and then come back. This will help you to get used to the mechanics of treadmill running which are

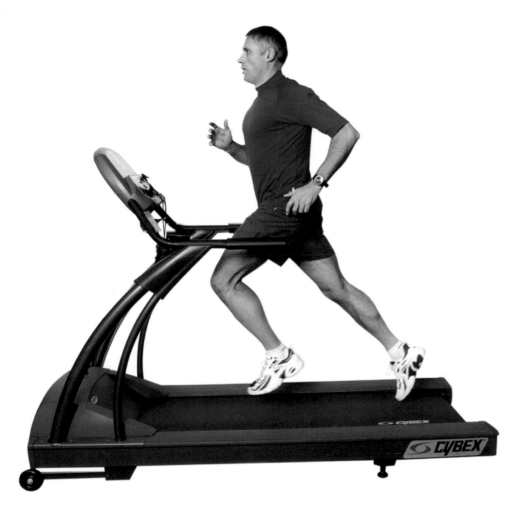

subtly different to road running (as your supporting leg is pulled behind you by the belt rather than you propelling your body over the top of it).

You will find various programme options including inclines and declines. Decline running will assist with your leg speed, but if you are overweight and out of condition stick with the 0% or 1% setting for several weeks (1% is said by most treadmill manufacturers to be the equivalent of flat road running as it compensates for the lack of wind resistance you obviously encounter in the gym) otherwise you could end up with lots of knee problems. If you are doing steep inclines and are overweight you are risking lower back problems as you end up stooping over the machine too much. Basically, just be sensible; because it's an indoor machine and is fixed to the floor doesn't mean it won't reproduce all the problems you would encounter if you ran out of your front door and flat out up the nearest hill without a proper warm-up.

It's the same with the stepper machine. Time and time again I see people climb on to a stepper and immediately work out at far too high an intensity. Remember, gaining fitness is largely about how long you can spend in an activity, it's not about getting on a machine and blasting for ten to fifteen minutes – yes that can improve your fitness, but it's very short-lived. The aim is to endure the activity at a low intensity rather than get on a machine for a quick ten-minute fix. As your endurance improves at the low intensity then, periodically, you can set yourself a five or ten-minute challenge, which is a very useful way to determine where you are at.

You will also see that most machines have a number of pre-set programmes, often called things like 'fat-burn, 'mountain' and 'random', which are designed, by increasing/decreasing the resistance or raising/lowering the inclination of the treadmill, to mimic the cardiovascular effects of variable terrains found during road running or hiking. I find these can be quite motivational – setting useful challenges and offering a degree of variation. But I would urge you to be careful if you find their use becoming your regular thing at the gym. You are going to reach a point where there's little control over your performance on the equipment and it will develop into nothing much more than 'turn up and challenge the machine' sessions with no reference to your structured training plan. Basically you will plateau off, become disillusioned by it all and start going backwards. The best way to avoid this is to base your training on a sensible diet of steady state endurance sessions that you can vary from time to time with intervals, random or mountain programmes. This way you will be keeping your body on its toes with varied training stimuli rather than getting into a training rut.

In summary, you need to bring an educated approach to these machines, making sure you are in full control of technique; I definitely think that the novice user should be able to say 'I could go a bit quicker'. Many times I have seen people pushing it with that fixed, not to say demented, stare and a horribly ragged, fatigued running style, with no idea that they are effectively out of control. My concern has less to do with seeing them fall off, rather the worry is the unnecessary and potentially dangerous stresses they are putting on vulnerable parts of the body. Remember, unlike the road or the hiking trail, the machine's platform is moving and will only slow down when you choose to slow the machine down – which is fantastic for holding a controlled steady state pace but potentially disastrous if you need to pull up in a hurry! It's worth knowing that even for top runners who do laboratory assessments at maximum pace on the treadmill, sports scientists will often put a mattress behind the machine just in case the athlete should lose pace and get chucked off the back!

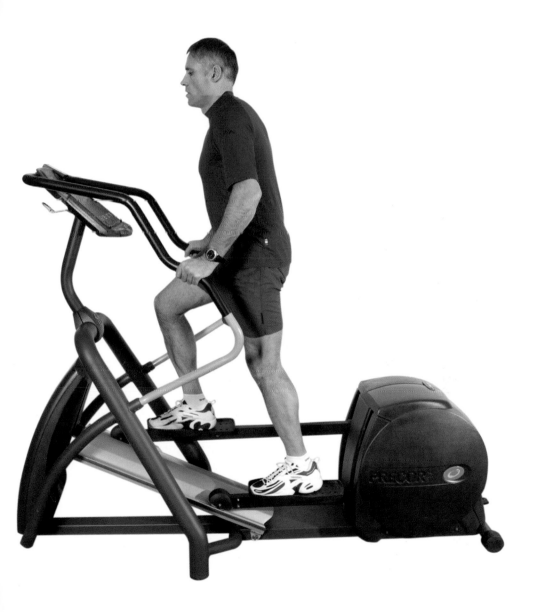

Core stability and functional training

- Supine bridge • Kneeling position • Roll-out
- Press-up • Superman and pendulum roll
- Back extension • F1 driver

WHEN I USE THE TERM 'CORE' stability, I am talking about that part of your body which lies between your neck and the tops of your thighs and which includes the trunk, lower back and hips.

In many sports there is a tendency to focus on the peripheries: a tennis player is always aware of his or her arm and shoulder; footballers, not unnaturally, tend to be fixated on their legs. But British mountain bike champion Oli Beckingsale or the members of the GB Rowing Team have all learnt that core strength is essential for generating explosive power in the limbs. Martial arts performers have long realised this; equally yoga concentrates on working the core area of the body. Core stability is vital for this whole range of activities, from extreme energy to serene control.

When I was a Marine, my core strength initially let me down, even though at the time I thought it was my arms. When I joined up, I could run and canoe well, but on what seemed a straightforward rope-climbing exercise I found that I was having difficulty bringing my legs up the rope. The reason was that my core strength was too weak for me to hold a strong static contraction, which stopped me being able to lift my legs up with my body held away from the rope and made me fatigue really quickly. I reckon that if I had spent some time working on the core region I could have got on much better

with the rope climbing, even though I was never super-strong in my arms.

Core conditioning will improve the basic condition of your muscles. If you've just been asked to play in a five-a-side soccer match, your brain may make you think you can still produce the skills you had fifteen years ago and that you can still turn on a sixpence. Unfortunately the conditioning of your core area might not support this kind of aggressive turn – and suddenly your groin's gone. Core stability work will help to bring those muscles back to the level of performance of years ago. Even at a comparatively modest level of performance it can give you an extra edge and provide you with an insurance policy against injury.

I really became aware of the importance of core stability when I started doing some serious K1 marathon kayaking. In this sport, balance is crucial, and during my first training session I found that the boat felt very unstable – so much so that my training partner and coach told me just to leave the boat on the shore and swim up and down the river instead, because that would save us having to empty the water out of the kayak every ten minutes!

Even though I thought I had pretty good general balance, I was very twitchy when I was sitting in the kayak. I realised that, like rowing, it is a sport that looks, from the outside, to be all about the arms, but it actually places a high level of emphasis

Without a strong core it doesn't matter how strong your arms and legs are – it's like applying pressure to a wobbly jelly.

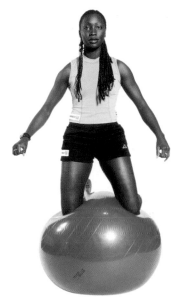

on core stability. Once you have acquired your basic balance, the trick is to keep everything over the centre line of the kayak. As the blade enters the water, you press down on the footrest with a slightly bent leg – it feels like cycling, and in fact 'cycling' is the term kayakers use to describe it. Once your foot is pressed down, everything is locked into your core. You drive the blade into water like a stake, and then, as if you were on rollerskates pulling yourself past a lamppost, the action is a rotation of trunk, not pulling with your arms at all. With the hands gripping the blade, and the feet on the leg bar, there is a triangle of dynamic activity that really works out the hip flexor and core area. From that you can see that a soft core region = loss of power transfer = inefficiency and fatigue. I wonder how many of you think about the subtleties of your own sports in this way?

When I went home after that session, my shoulders felt stiff, which was fine, but when I woke up the next day, I could really feel the effect the training session had had on my hip flexors and core area. I couldn't even sit up in bed. It was as if I'd had a couple of concrete slabs smashed on my stomach. But when I did some running after a few weeks of K1 training, I could see a definite improvement, and I realised just how strong I had become in my core area. It brought home to me how important core conditioning is – especially now that I am in my mid-40s – and also why coaches and physios at the highest level put so much attention on the core: firstly because so much energy can be

generated from that area, and also as an insurance policy against injury. Working with Jenson Button, I know that he really gains a great deal out of our early morning hikes with ski poles up steep gradients and rough terrain, which really works his core region. Jenson is very aware of the long-term benefits for his core area – and the bonus for his lower back during the rigours of the next Grand Prix.

For these reasons, and for all kinds of training, you should aim to incorporate core stability work in your programme. It is subtle work, neither overly hard nor aggressive, but you will find that the benefits are substantial.

One term that has recently come into vogue and is highly related to training the core region, and which you might well hear being bandied about by fitness professionals, is 'functional training'. What does 'functional training' mean?

In my day in the Marines the concept of physiotherapy was totally unknown. The PTIs just used to shout, 'Keep going, it's only broken!'

It's essentially a phrase taken from the world of physiotherapy, and means any exercise that gets a muscle 'functioning' again – possibly after a stroke, an injury or to correct postural or technical faults in sport. It could be something quite simple: a repetitive movement while lying on a couch, a subtle movement designed to work on a muscle imbalance, develop a specific muscle group after a layoff or concentrate on a particular weakness.

'Functional training' is also often used to describe a slightly unconventional or adapted exercise that incorporates an element of core control or simulates a sporting movement. For instance, a simple squat might be performed on an unstable platform to increase core strength in the lower back region and help develop balance – in this way it becomes a 'functional exercise'.

Functional training is essentially about going back to basics, and the kind of exercises we're going to be looking at in the next section are very much along the same lines: subtle exercises that have both an overall and specific impact on the way your body functions. There's nothing particularly revolutionary about this approach – 'functional training' just happens to be the current buzzword for it – but you'll find that these sorts of exercises are as effective as ever.

Modern physiotherapists have had a major influence on the way that their work can complement sports. If you go to watch the GB Rowing Team training, you will find a team of physios working closely with them. Time was that a physio used to be a man with an aerosol and a magic sponge (to a certain extent, that is still true in some amateur sports).

Thankfully, sport is slowly emerging from those Dark Ages. In rugby, the England team of twenty years ago never really did any specific functional or core stability work (unless there's a functional element involved in staggering in the bar after a few pints!). Now it forms an essential part of their preparation, whether that's generating the power to kick a 50-metre penalty, or driving into a scrum where all the strength comes from contracting the core to fix the legs solidly and propel as much energy as possible through the body into the scrum.

Most of the exercises in this section involve the Swiss physio ball, or the exercise ball as it's more generally known. Originally used, as the name suggests, in Switzerland in the 1950s, the ball formed part of a physiotherapy programme to help the posture and mobility of children with cerebral palsy. The fitness industry latched onto the exercise ball in the late 1990s and turned it into something of a gimmick. This doesn't make them useless, far from it, but you need to understand the way that they can help you. Don't just roll around on them or copy other people in the gym; get some quality tuition to get the most out of them. And don't be fooled by the fact that some of these exercises look easy. An exercise like the one shown on page 109, which involves kneeling on an exercise ball and sucking in your stomach with your feet off the floor, is made up of controlled, small movements, but your core muscles are really working. Fighting to keep your balance on the ball means those muscles are having to adjust all the time. Only a quarter of an hour of this kind of balancing starts recruiting and employing muscle fibres that may not have been used for a very long time.

Doing anything that is performed on an unstable surface can be good for your core: windsurfing, running across an uneven field, skiing off piste. Don't think that it has to be limited to the selection of Swiss ball exercises shown on the next few pages.

My son Gregg uses a tummy wheel to build up his hip flexibility for his butterfly stroke. People think it's a bit odd but it does his core strength no end of good and complements his sport brilliantly.

Some of the core stability exercises in this section are not just for that region; they help work out much of the rest of the body as well. It is about reducing the weakest link – once your core is getting strong, you need to work simultaneously on the other parts of your body; but if you don't work on your core, you will definitely find that the quality of your overall performance is reduced.

Think of these exercises as complementary to your programme, rather than a separate session. You complement a training session by doing some exercises before and after the main workout. If you are very unfit, or are returning after injury, you could start off with a session entirely made up of these exercises and doing so will bring you on quite rapidly, but as soon as possible move on to a broader programme. They should be the spices that enhance the flavour of the cake, not the cake itself.

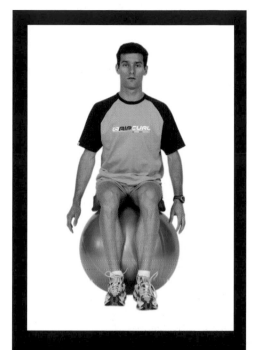

To get used to the feel of working with the exercise ball, you can start by sitting on an appropriate ball (see the sizing chart over the page) with a good upright posture. Do be careful – you are on an unstable piece of equipment and make sure you can fall without hitting an object or a hard floor. Use a mat and move the furniture. When you are doing these exercises be sure that you make use of a mirror, if one is available, to check that your form and your shape during each exercise is correct. As you should have picked up from me by now, the quality with which any exercise is performed is the most crucial factor above all else. Learn to critique yourself and your technique in the mirror, especially when using the exercise ball.

Supine bridge position

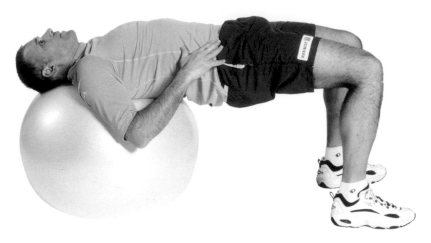

This is a postural position that works all the muscles in the core region, including the abs, transverse abs and lumbar region, and which also works the hips, glutes and quads statically. Like the exercise opposite it looks easy but holding the position accurately is the main thing. The supine position is a basic bridge; to get into the position, start by sitting on the ball and then walking your feet out until your knees are flexed at an angle of 90 degrees and your shoulder blades are in contact with the ball. Remember to keep your hips up – don't sag or over-arch in the middle.

Start off by trying to hold this position accurately for 5 or 10 seconds and build up the length of time as you become stronger and/or more proficient. A tough variation (shown below) is to lift one leg off the floor. This puts you in a very unstable position and to do this properly without dropping the hips or wobbling around takes a great deal of practice.

HEIGHT CHART
(APPLIES TO ALL EXERCISES)

Swiss ball size	Height range
45cm	5ft and under
55cm	5ft 1in to 5ft 7in
65cm	5ft 8in to 6ft
75cm	6ft 1in to 6ft 3in
85cm	6ft 4in and over

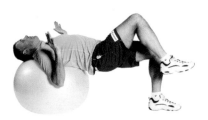

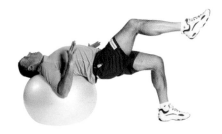

Kneeling position
and variation

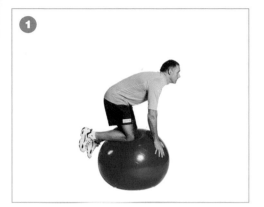

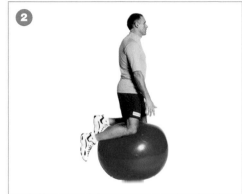

This exercise looks deceptively simple, but straightaway you will feel how hard your muscles are working. The kneeling position on a ball requires excellent balance and works most of your muscles through the thighs, buttocks, core region and, to a certain extent, the upper body.

The most difficult part of this exercise is getting or finding your balance point on the ball. As you can see in photo 1 above, you start off by placing your knees and the tops of your shins on the centre of the ball with your hands placed towards the front to stop you falling flat on your face.

As you feel your balance in this initial position improving, gradually rise up by pushing your hips slightly forwards and your arms down by your sides – then hold this position. Use a mirror or partner to maintain good posture, keeping your hips well forward and your shoulders held back. When you get as good at balancing on the ball as those circus elephants you can add a few variations such as being passed a light medicine ball, moving it from hand to hand and eventually having someone else throw a ball to you, which, in turn, you can throw back to them at a range of heights and angles.

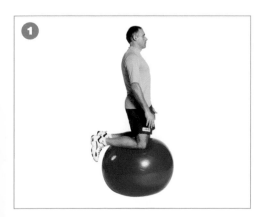

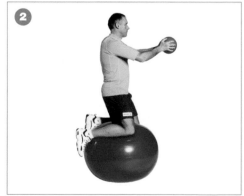

Roll-out and press-up

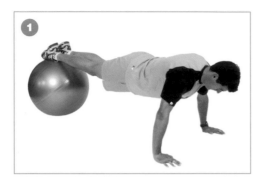

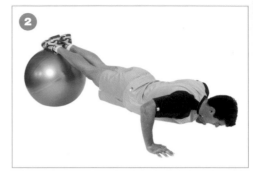

Start by kneeling over the ball with it tucked into your stomach. Bring your feet together and walk out on your hands while rolling the ball to your shins. By now you should be taking most of your body weight through your arms and your arms will be more or less straight (photo 1). From there do a press-up making sure all the time you keep your body flat; don't sag or arch.

There are a couple of variations which you can use once you have mastered the initial technique of rolling out and moving into the press-up. Either roll out, complete a press-up and roll back before repeating the movement or, having rolled out, perform several press-ups. Always finish the exercise by rolling back to the start position – don't just drop your legs off the side of the ball.

Increase the difficulty by rolling out from the ball which is resting against your shins to the tips of your toes – this is really hard.

Unlike a normal floor press-up, when you use the Swiss ball your core region has to stabilise the power generated by your arms and chest, otherwise the ball (and you) will go all over the place. This is a really good core conditioning exercise, and it has the added bonus of conditioning your arms and chest.

You can also turn the exercise around and use the ball to work against. As in photos 3 and 4 below you can perform a press-up while using the ball as an unstable platform. This is terrific for shoulder stability; when starting off you might find it easier to place the ball in a corner of the room to stop it moving about too much.

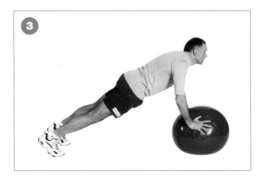

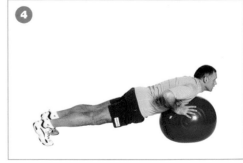

Superman
and pendulum roll

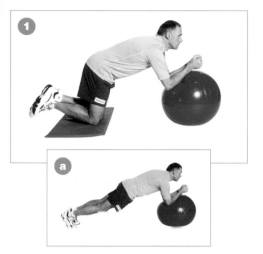

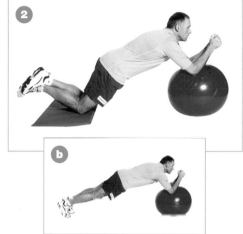

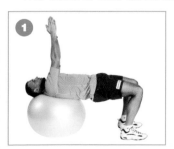

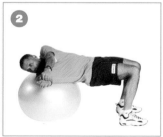

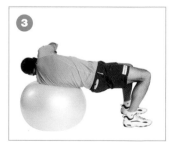

The Superman is so-called because it looks like a superhero flying into action. This is a real toughie, which really works your abs (an alternative to crunches) and is good for shoulder stability. The two variations shown get progressively harder.

For the first exercise, start in a kneeling position with your elbows and forearms on the ball; the ball should be just in front of you. Then roll out onto the points of your elbows slowly and in a controlled way. Hold the position for a couple of seconds and then roll back. Go on and try it; feel how difficult it is to complete the action – you'll feel it all the way up your trunk and especially in the abs.

The second and advanced variation (photos a and b) applies the same principles. Start by balancing on your toes and with straight legs rather than on your knees.

The pendulum roll (below) is another exercise for balance and coordination and brings in trunk rotations which work the obliques. The start position is the same as the supine position (on page 108) only this time the arms are held at 90 degrees (vertically) to the body, and the exercise is to roll your shoulders across the ball twisting through the mid section in a slow, controlled way – no arching or sagging – from one side to the other. You can also hold a very light weight as you improve.

Back extension

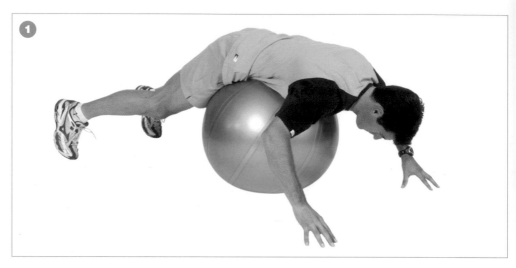

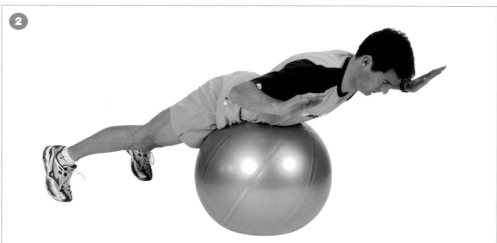

Back extensions (not hair extensions!) are often performed incorrectly with a lot of people hyperextending their back far too vigorously. What I mean by this is over-arching the back which is a recipe for back injury. You should ideally move from a flexed position at the waist to only a very small degree of extension past a flat back.

Look at Mark Webber in these photos and you can see how he maintains a nice neutral head position throughout and works in a safe range of movement. Hyperextension is used only when training for very specific sports like gymnastics where working with an exaggerated range of motion is an essential performance factor.

F1 driver

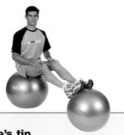

This is an exercise that has evolved from working with single-seat racing drivers and kayakers, who have different needs but who sit in very similar positions to practise their sports.

The benefit for the racing drivers, who are strapped into their seated position when in the car, is the conditioning of their postural muscles (the lumbar region of the back and the hip flexors, for example) whereas the kayakers, who maintain their position in the kayak through balance and coordination skills, benefit from practising the balance aspects.

The activity can also be adapted by using a weighted disk as a pretend steering wheel to work the shoulders and arms – or a kayaker might hold his or her paddle.

Bernie's tip
Like K1 paddling, this exercise is very good for balance. I developed it with Jenson Button and Mark Webber to create a strong core. Once you have good balance you can use a 5kg weight for the steering wheel.

The hardest part of this exercise is getting into the position. Start by sitting on the larger of the two Swiss balls and ask someone to position the smaller one for your feet. You might want them to hold onto it for a while as you get your balance. Now hold the position using the mirror for good posture – and remember, don't come off into the fireplace while you're coming through the chicane!

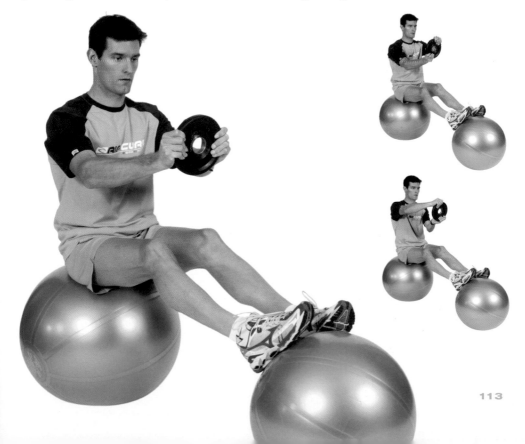

Compound exercises

- **Deadlift • Squat • Squat and curl**
- **Bench press • Push press or jerk**

IN THIS SECTION I HAVE SELECTED five key exercises to examine in detail because they can be used as the main components in a variety of strength and conditioning programmes. Between them they cover virtually every muscle group in the body and use a number of techniques that are vital in more advanced weightlifting.

You will see that all of these exercises use only free weights – i.e. they are not machine-based. This is important because their patterns of movement are more applicable to sporting situations; in addition, the exercises can be done anywhere that has some basic weights and bars.

Those of you who have a more advanced background in strength training may be wondering why I have not included Olympic lifts such as the clean and jerk or the snatch in this section. These represent the ultimate in strength and power training but technically are incredibly complex, requiring one-to-one coaching and a lot of practice to perfect. However, some of the exercises here do contain elements of those techniques and can help to develop the basic conditioning and movement patterns which will help you move on to the next level. Just remember you should get proper instruction for this so that you don't end up feeling sorry for yourself sitting in A&E in your vest and shorts.

The deadlift is a cracking exercise to start with. It uses nearly all of the muscles in the body and is fantastic for the legs and back. If you follow the technique guidelines on pages 116–117 you will feel yourself getting stronger for any sort of lifting and bending activities (you know, the important ones, like heaving a crate of beer out of a supermarket trolley). This is a top-end core stability workout which will really let you know that you've done some work the day after your first session! Take it easy for the first few sets, otherwise you'll wake up wondering if you got run over by a bus in your sleep. Deadlifts also generate a lot of grip strength as you'll probably be heaving some pretty big weights around when you get going. Don't be afraid to experiment with grip styles (see page 116) to help cope with this.

The squat is another exercise that builds great core stability because this time you are moving unsupported with a heavy weight balanced high above your centre of gravity. Start off with moderate loading and pay attention to immaculate technique (pages 118–119) to avoid injuries. Squats develop power and strength from the legs and hips and so are a vital part of training for huge numbers of sportspeople, because a large part of most activities require us to generate power from the floor via our feet and legs. Squats are much more effective than just doing machine leg presses, say, because of all the extra muscles you recruit just standing there with the bar on your shoulders. You will find that you will develop the ability to transfer the strength you evolve into your sport or your daily activities. Above all don't be afraid of squats – they're not bad for your knees, as many people will have you believe, as long as you do them correctly; the potential benefits for your improved strength are massive.

The squat and curl (pages 120–121) is a clever variation on the squat which I learnt from working with top rowers. If you think about it, this exercise pretty much replicates the rowing motion in a vertical rather than a horizontal plane, and so it is very relevant for that sport.

The trick with the squat and curl is to learn to use the momentum generated by the drive up in the legs from the squat position to help initiate the curl. This not only teaches the neuromuscular system to transfer power effectively from your legs through the body to your arms (a must-have quality in most sports) but allows you to overload the arms with larger weights than you would usually use for a straight curl. Put it this way: if I only had 40 minutes to get a quick strength workout in the gym I'd much rather do a set of squat and curls than spend twice as long doing separate sets of both.

The bench press has been included in this section because it is a major exercise in many people's strength training and I feel it is important to highlight how to do it safely and properly. It complements the other exercises here by adding a chest and arms emphasis to the selection, and it is very specific to some sports such as rugby,

where you need to hand off an opponent with a well-timed shove. Just try not to join the 'how much can you bench press?' club by spending half your training time on this exercise, unless you fancy getting that top-heavy look that many amateur meatheads seem to perfect!

The push press or jerk (pages 124–125) is a combination exercise which is a bit like the squat and curl, but which brings into play a great 'kinetic chain' – excuse the fancy terminology – as you work right from the calves up to the arms and shoulders. It is obviously the last phase of a 'clean and jerk' movement although you can start it from the chest by picking the bar off a chest-high rack instead of flipping up from the floor. This is another favourite of mine as it also uses the neuromuscular element of transferring power from your legs through the entire body. If you get it right you can press far more weight above your head than by using your shoulders alone. In fact top weightlifters will jerk up to three times their body weight in training! Use it as a precursor to getting into Olympic-style lifting or as a general conditioning exercise for your sport. It is spot-on for throwing events like shot put as it has similar movement patterns, recruiting fibres from feet to fingertips.

You can use one or more of these exercises to complement an efficient total body workout if you've only got your lunch break to train in. Or you can use them to enhance a crucial part of your sport performance. As I keep saying, technique is everything, though. Leave your ego at home – start with the smaller weights and build up gradually.

The deadlift

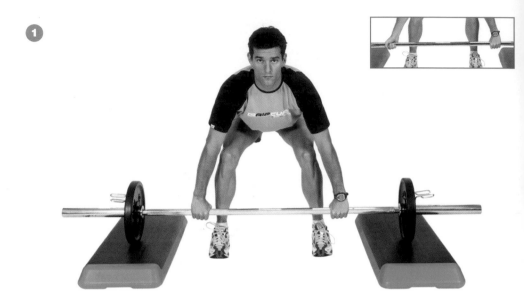

Standing behind the bar, grasping it as shown, with your feet about shoulder width apart, bend your knees, bringing your thighs to roughly parallel with the floor and making sure you keep your back flat. The grip on the bar can be overhand, although for very heavy weights some people prefer one hand over and one under as shown in the inset picture.

The first movement is to straighten the legs at the knee; you'll need to tighten your abs and make sure you keep your back straight – otherwise you run the risk of possible injury – as the bar moves up towards your knees. Next, extend your trunk, keeping your arms straight by your side. To complete the movement push your hips forward: the bar should be resting on your upper thighs. From here lower the weight to the floor; do not just flex the back to do this, but use your knees in a smooth, controlled movement

With extremely heavy weights you might see experienced weightlifters simply drop the weight at the completion of the lift. This is because the eccentric movement

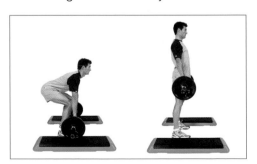

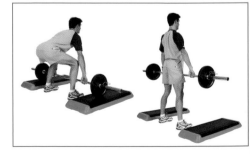

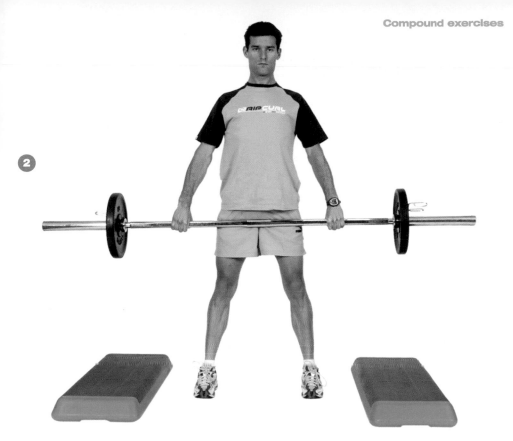

2

(i.e. the return movement) places a greater load on the back and consequently the risk of injury is high.

The deadlift is one of the few exercises that truly works nearly every single muscle in the body to some degree or another.

The 'stiff leg deadlift' is a variation which places greater emphasis on the hips, buttocks and thighs. It also requires good flexibility in the hamstrings to execute it properly. The action is very similar to the normal deadlift but as shown below, the feet are brought slightly closer together and your legs are only very subtly flexed at the knee – they are essentially straight but with soft knees. There is no real need to lock the legs. This variation is quite stressful in the lumbar region of the back, and is a technically demanding exercise. It should be approached with caution and using sensible loading.

The deadlift is a core exercise in strength conditioning employed by a range of athletes and sportspeople as part of any general strength-conditioning exercise. It is a fantastic all-rounder.

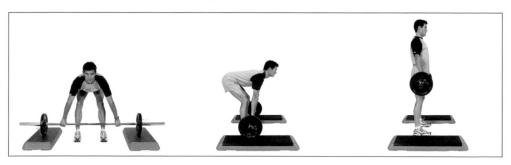

The squat

The squat looks familiar as it's a classic weightlifting move, but just because you recognise it, you shouldn't underestimate how technical an exercise it is, and how carefully you need to prepare for it. This is not something you can watch on *The World's Strongest Man*, when somebody lifts two Minis with the help of an A frame, and then try at home.

So let's start with the technique. We need to begin by learning the correct movement patterns, so that all the muscles involved know what they are supposed to be doing and in what order – this is called neuromuscular training.

A good way to start this is by using a broomstick or lightweight body bar in place of the full Olympic bar (which you can see being used by Mark Webber in the photographs). This gets your whole body into the correct position without unnecessary loading.

The basic squat position starts with the feet just under shoulder width apart and toes ever so slightly pointed out rather than completely straight (see photos).

Squat down keeping your upper body vertical, heels on the floor and the core region contracted; you should feel as if you are about to sit down on a low bench. Keeping the heels on the floor throughout the exercise is crucial and can be quite challenging at first, so make sure you concentrate on this aspect of the technique. There is no need to drop lower than the point at which your thighs are parallel with the floor. Powerlifters often go much lower, but to do so can take years of training and is, in any case, both very stressful on the knees and of negligible benefit for most of us.

From the low position now stand up, pressing through the heels. Pressing through the heels reduces the likelihood of rising up on your toes, and puts the emphasis on the quadriceps and glutes, rather than the calves, which are not the primary target in this exercise.

The squat is a key lift for many sports people as it recruits ankle, knee and hip extensors (in that order), which is a common series in all sorts of sports. Basically, any activity where you apply force

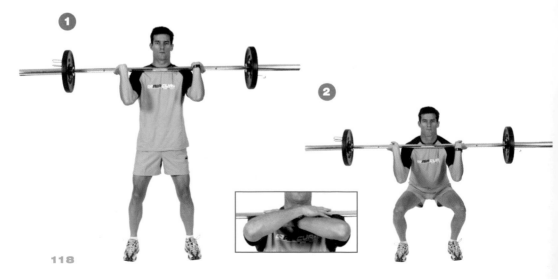

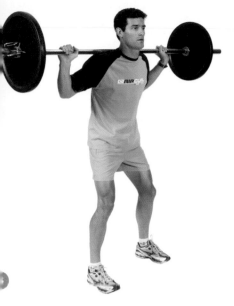

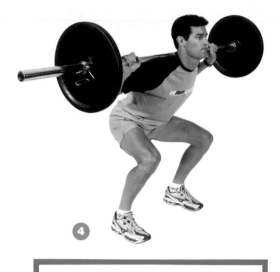

(4)

to the ground for jumping and running will benefit from strong extensors as will sports like cycling and rowing where the force is applied to the apparatus by the legs.

When you've got the technique sorted with a broomstick, the serious ironmongery awaits, but be sure (at the risk of repeating myself) to start steadily and build up to heavier weights gradually. Take note of the tip box (right) and use a proper rack, to lift the bar from and return it to, during each set. Also note that with the weight up high on your upper back, your trunk is very vulnerable – you have been warned!

Incidentally, the reason a lot of guys wear a belt whilst squatting is not, as many people think, to support the lower back but to give something external to strain against and to increase the air pressure in the trunk. This supports the lumbar region by making the core solid.

The basic squat involves holding the bar across the trapezius muscles behind the head (note: not across the neck), however one variation (the front squat) is to shift the bar onto the chest as shown in photos 3 and 4. The front squat places more emphasis on the quads and reduces the

Always use a proper weight rack to pick up and return the weights to. Take the time to get the height set right too – after 10 reps of 100kg you don't want to have to climb on your tiptoes to put the bar back on a rack that is too high.

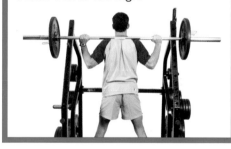

emphasis on the glutes. You may find that you cannot lift quite as much weight during the front squat, so bear that in mind when loading up the bar. It also requires excellent lower back strength so be careful when you try this variation for the first time.

The squat is, quite correctly, a key exercise in most strength training programmes – get it right and it will deliver considerable improvement in your basic lower body strength. Don't be afraid of it – just take the time to get your technique refined before you hit the heavy stuff.

The squat and curl

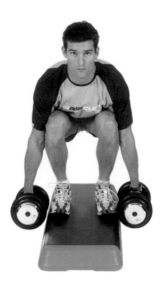

The squat and curl is not widely used, but is an excellent combination exercise for many sports, particularly rowing.

Stand with your arms by your sides, palms facing inwards, feet shoulder width apart, and lower yourself into a squat posi-

tion with your thighs parallel to the floor, heels flat and back straight. The power for the movement is initiated through the legs as they extend (and you move up); then your lower back muscles come into play as they extend your trunk. The arms com-

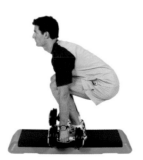
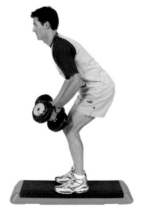

2

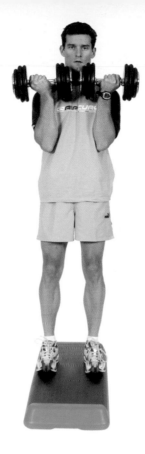

plete the movement with the biceps doing most of the work. As you can see, even a weedy F1 driver like Mark Webber can curl quite respectable dumbbells using the momentum generated by the legs and the back, if his technique is good. You should be able to squat and curl more than you can curl alone. Remember to keep a flat back (don't arch over) in the initial squat. You may also find you need to stand on a box or platform to stop the weights resting on the floor at the start of the movement.

3

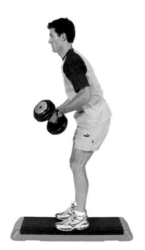

4

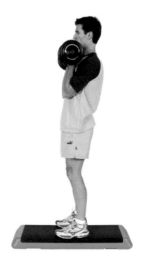

The bench press

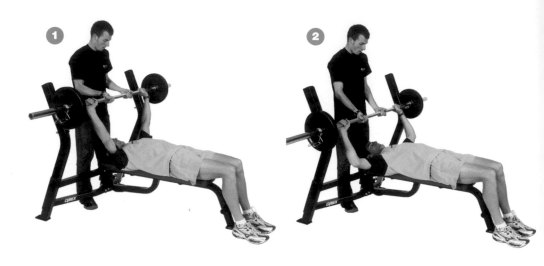

The bench press is an exercise which is central to a lot of people's strength and conditioning programmes.

The standard bench press is a chest and arm exercise that works the pecs and triceps primarily, with contributions from the deltoids and subscapularis amongst others.

To get the maximum benefit from your benching, avoid falling into the trap of lifting massive weights really slowly just to impress your mates. The exercise done properly is a combination of both speed and a full range of movement – and you should be aiming to optimise both.

The basic hand position for the bench press – and probably the strongest position for most people – is set slightly wider than the shoulders. Make sure that the spacing of your hands is even by using the knurl grips on the bar. This uses the optimum combination of mechanical advantage and force generation from the muscle. If you bring in a narrow grip this enhances the contribution of the triceps as you are lifting the bar by extending the arms at the elbow.

If you use an exaggerated wide grip that leaves the arms a lot straighter, the pectorals are used to a greater extent.

Your feet should be flat on the floor for good stability; try to keep your back flat with a minimum of arching. The bar should be across the top of the chest, virtually touching it, and the elbows sunk below the level of the bench (see photo 3). Breathe in as you lower the bar to your chest, hold your breath, then exhale explosively on completion of the movement. Do not breathe out too early as the whole purpose of holding your breath is to increase intra-thoracic pressure which stabilises your core region, protects it from injury and provides a solid base to support your arms (this, by the way, is known as the Valsalva manoeuvre and is a natural reflex and what happens automatically when you try to pick up a heavy suitcase). Fully straighten your arms; then lower the weight with controlled speed back to the start position within a few millimetres of the chest. It is important to complete a full range of motion.

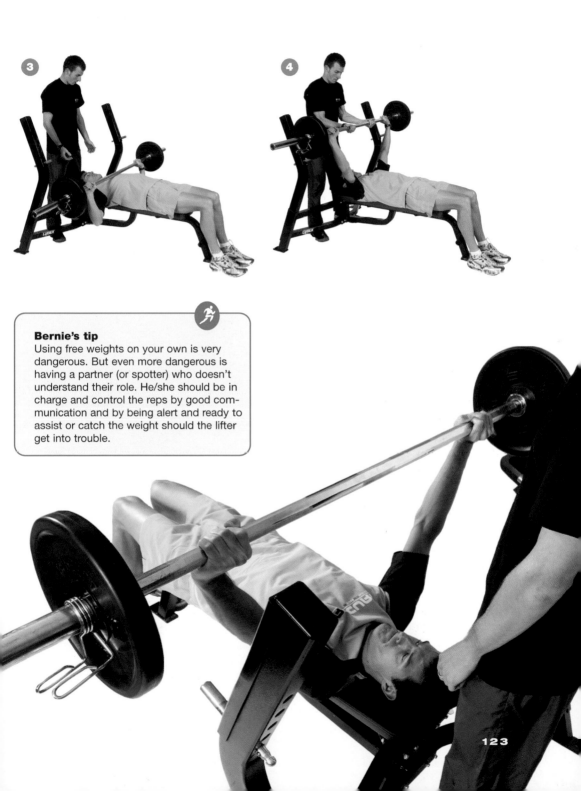

Bernie's tip

Using free weights on your own is very dangerous. But even more dangerous is having a partner (or spotter) who doesn't understand their role. He/she should be in charge and control the reps by good communication and by being alert and ready to assist or catch the weight should the lifter get into trouble.

The push press
(also known as the jerk)

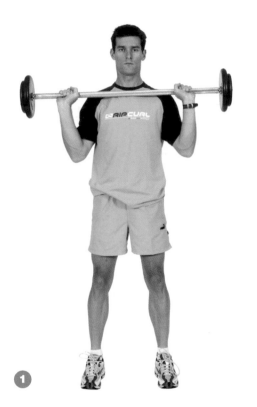

1

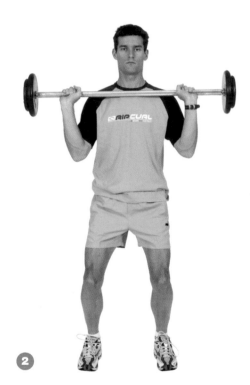

2

Don't confuse the push press with the straightforward shoulder press. The push press is a much more dynamic exercise and uses the power of the legs as well as the shoulders to lift the weight.

It is sometimes referred to as a jerk as in the 'clean and jerk' performed by Olympic weightlifters. The idea is to lift a significantly heavier weight than you would during a shoulder press. Begin the

movement with a slight bending of the knees and immediately extend the knees powerfully to get the weight moving vertically as if you are jumping in the air. Extend your arms while pressing the weight upwards to a fully extended position. Depending on the weight you are using, you might rise up on your toes. As you lower the weight to its starting position, bend the knees slightly again to

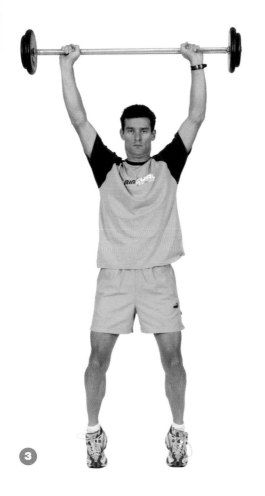

3

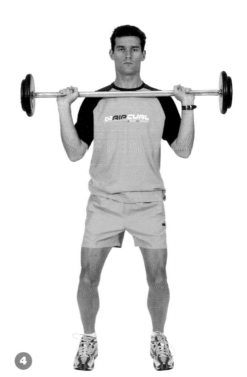

4

absorb the impact. Settle into a fully recovered starting position before you repeat the movement.

This is an extremely quick movement which should be performed explosively. However, you will get out of rhythm if you try to do push presses on a speed circuit. It is designed to increase the explosive power of your body and to improve coordination and muscle recruitment, and it is a fairly technical exercise. When you think about it, most sporting activities require the coordination of movement to transfer power from a static position (the ground, say, if you are a shot putter) out to the peripheries.

The push press teaches your body how to transfer power effectively from your legs to the tips of your fingers: invaluable in a tennis serve, for example.

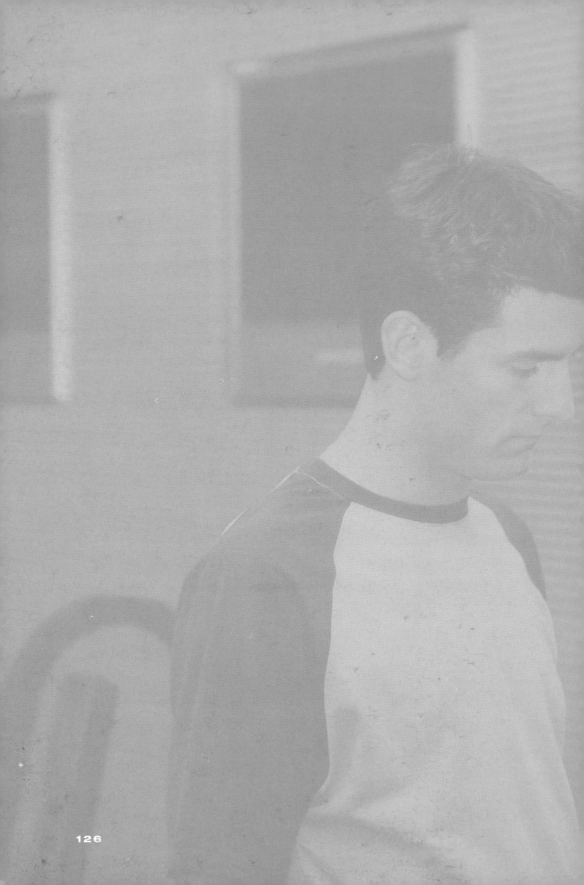

The muscle groups

I've got to be honest, I never got too excited in my early days of training as a young cross-country skier about strength training, circuit sessions or any other stuff we got up to in the gym. Remember my roots are in an era when most gyms were underground, rough and ready basements. In these places, only the most dedicated strength and power athletes and body builders worked out using basic free weights and you could probably have found many unidentified organisms flourishing in the corner of the changing rooms. Nowadays it's a bit different though!

The gyms we are all used to now are full of machines and equipment that even I don't always instantly recognise. Although this has made the fitness club a much more versatile, safer and more accessible environment for most of us to train in, you still need a sound knowledge of the basics of good exercise techniques and principles of training to get the most out of them.

I have learnt the value of gym based training over the last twenty-five years though, and these days have a more open mind about the benefits of the specific conditioning that can be achieved with knowledge and hard work in the indoor environment. Getting a bit older has taught me about the need to stave off some of the effects of ageing such as atrophy in the muscles (basically wasting away slowly) and the loss of flexibility and range of movement due to breakdown of the elastic components of the muscle tissue, and how some tailored gym work can help with this. I've also worked with sports where a great percentage of training time is spent on strength and conditioning (F1, rugby and rowing) and have grown to appreciate the importance of getting this training right to optimise performance out in the real world of modern sport.

The following sections are broken down into regions of the body to help you understand a few fundamental basics of your own anatomy and a series of exercises related to each region is discussed. I'll show you some appropriate techniques and give you ideas on how to train different areas for different activities. The exercise lists are not supposed to be exhaustive by any means but show a combination of the most common ones and some of my personal favourites.

What I'd like you to do is get to understand some of the subtleties of the exercises I've highlighted and arm yourself with some sound knowledge before you go off to the gym and believe everything you see and hear down there. I'm often horrified by what I see in the health club environment these days. The ignorance about technique is frightening, as is people's reluctance to seek out decent advice or to ask what they think might be seen as 'a dumb question' – in fact, those are often the most important questions. Take responsibility for the quality of your own training and you'll see the payback – I'll guarantee that. So read on and make sure that you're paying attention!

The shoulders

- **Shoulder press** • **Dumbbell raises**
- **Rotator cuff rotation**
- **Upright row and shoulder shrugs**

MANY PEOPLE SPEND A LOT OF THEIR time concentrating on their arms and completely forget about working on their shoulders. The reason you need to think about your shoulders is that it's an extremely vulnerable part of your body. It is mobile, but does not have very much protection from injury. This is because the collar bone extends from your sternum – the breastbone – and holds the humerus, the upper arm bone, by one tiny joint. Effectively that's all there is holding your arm onto your body. So in sports where

there is a high level of physical contact and impact, like rugby, or where falls are commonplace, like soccer, the stronger the shoulder the better. And of course any event like the javelin or shot put, where throwing is important, will benefit from additional strength in the shoulder region.

Some sports also involve both a throwing action combined with the possibility of a high-impact injury. American football quarterbacks who get tackled with their arm cocked in the throwing position by a 20-stone linebacker are more than likely to

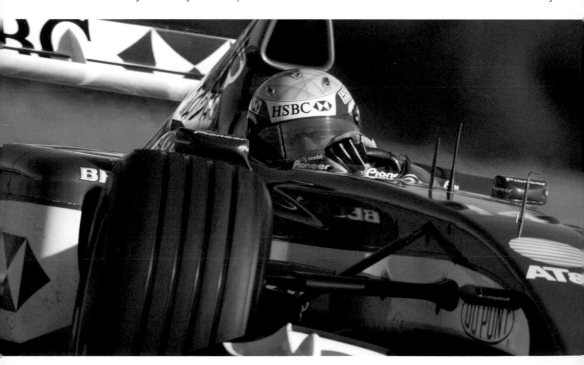

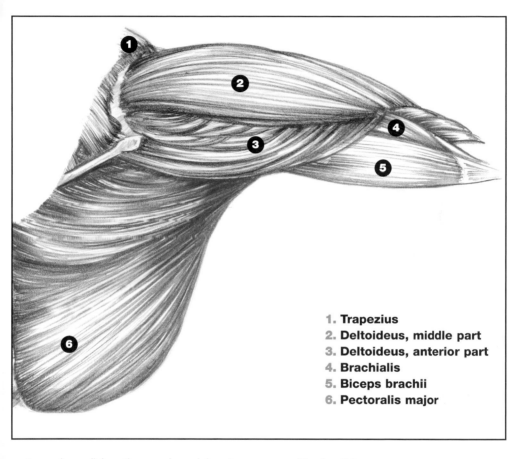

1. **Trapezius**
2. **Deltoideus, middle part**
3. **Deltoideus, anterior part**
4. **Brachialis**
5. **Biceps brachii**
6. **Pectoralis major**

get a serious dislocation, and any injury to the shoulder can cause long-term problems.

In this section we will be working on all aspects of the shoulder. Most of us are at least aware of the existence of the deltoids (the tulip-shaped group of three 'petal' muscles: the anterior, medial and posterior deltoids), but there are many deeper muscles beneath them which need to be conditioned as well. Sports like swimming, rowing, canoeing and cross-country skiing are tremendous for conditioning this area.

We may not aspire to the enormous shoulder strength of a gymnast performing the crucifix position on the rings, but nevertheless we can make sure that our own strength conditioning is vastly improved. In this section, you should really take notice of the combination exercises, which will give you a much better all-round effect, rather than just doing endless shoulder presses. Nevertheless, that's where we'll start.

Shoulder press

with barbell and dumbbell

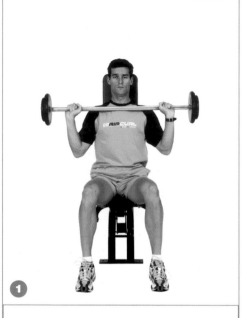

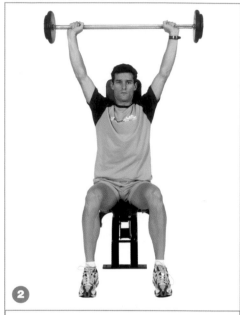

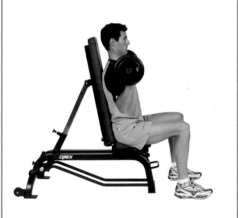

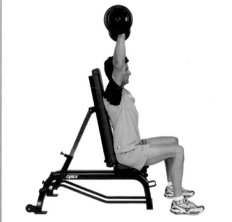

Bernie's tip

It is possible to do shoulder presses with the barbell starting off behind the neck – you've probably seen people doing this in the gym. I generally don't recommend this except at an advanced level, the reason being that the more difficult lifting angle can cause an impingement muscle injury, whereas the front position is more straightforward and certainly much less injury-prone.

You lift the barbell straight up in this exercise and it gets pretty close to your face. So watch out, big nose!

The shoulder press targets various muscles in the shoulder region including the anterior and medial deltoids, the upper pectorals, trapezius and the triceps, and the serratus anterior; it is probably the best known of all shoulder exercises. Some guys never do anything else, but that is really not such a great idea as you will only build up one aspect of your shoulders' range of movement. Try to use the press as part of an overall programme.

For the basic exercise sit on the bench (ideally with a back support), your posture upright and your feet flat on the floor to give you a good, wide base. Use an overhand grip on the bar of the barbell, with your hands slightly wider than your shoulders, and rest the bar on the upper part of your pecs, in front of your neck.

When you are set and balanced, you should be pressing the weight upwards in a straight vertical line and in one single movement, exhaling towards the top of the

lift. Keep your head fixed, looking straight forward. At the top avoid locking your arms out – you're not trying to win the gold medal in the Olympic weightlifting finals.

The actual lift off the chest will be quite hard initially, but you will find the second phase of the lift easier, simply because of your body's basic mechanical set-up. Hold your breath throughout the first phase, because this will stabilise your core region. It's the same thing you do instinctively when you pick up a heavy suitcase off the airport carousel.

You can also perform shoulder presses with dumbbells (photos below). This gives you the opportunity to use the arms alternately, working on your coordination, and also allowing you to work on the weaker arm.

Remember that you will tend to fatigue quite quickly doing shoulder presses since the muscles involved are not huge. So, as ever, take it easy, don't overstrain yourself.

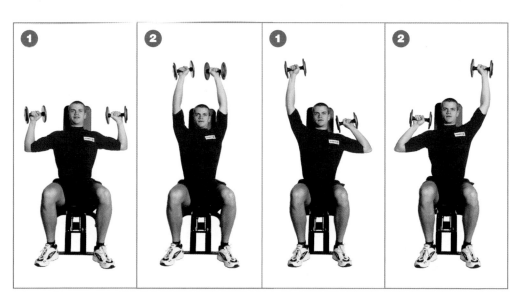

Dumbbell raises
Front raise, side lateral raises and dumbbell swing

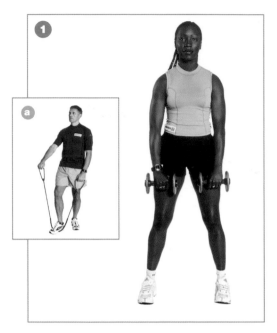

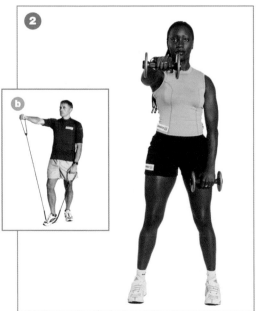

This group of exercises concentrates on the deltoids, but in a different motion than the shoulder press. The front lateral raise, for example, works the anterior and medial deltoids.These muscles come into play if you are lifting something with your arms fixed and your elbow level or higher than your hands (whereas if your elbow is lower than your hands you'll generally be using the biceps more by bending your arm).

I like to see anyone who is taking part in contact sports, throwing events or racquet sports spending time working on this exercise – it's another one of those insurance conditioning exercises which help prevent shoulder injuries.

So while these exercises might look less impressive than the shoulder press, they are vitally important. Don't underestimate their value. As you'll gather in the course of reading this book, I'm not a huge fan of those egotists who think that the more weight the better, just because it makes them look more macho. In my experience I've found that elite sportspeople achieve their goals by doing exercises like the ones on these two pages, using lower weights and more repetitions.

These dumbbell raises are quite similar, but they each involve a subtle but significant difference.

For the front lateral raises (left), hold the dumbbells with your palms down, feet shoulder width apart, your knees soft, and the weight in front of your thighs. Raise the weight with a straight arm until it's at 90 degrees to your body, exhaling as you reach the top of the lift. Then return the weight to the start position.

These exercises will strengthen you up to carry your mum's shopping bags for her.

The dumbbell swing (below) is a circuit exercise I discovered through my involvement in cross-country skiing. I used to put this into a circuit after press-ups and triceps dips, and imagined it would be an easy exercise. In fact, it's surprising how quickly it can fatigue you even with only a 2kg weight. Whereas the front and side lateral raises are stop and start, the dumbbell swing is a continuous motion without any pauses, swinging out to the side, out to the front and up and back – and continuous motion means continuous activity and energy. Try it and you'll see what I mean.

 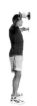 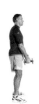   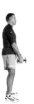

If you are arching your back, it means the weight you are using is too heavy. Don't cheat by using your back to flick the weight up.

Keep your body static and let the deltoids do all the work – that's what this exercise is for; leave your ego at home. You can also perform this exercise with a bungee cord to achieve the same effect (inset photos).

The bent-over side lateral raise (below) is a combination exercise which works all three deltoid muscles. A favourite variation of mine is to include a slight twist of the arm and hand when you get to the top of the movement (inset, picture 3). This uses the brachioradialis and is tougher than it looks. Try to keep the elbow high as you twist the dumbbell, imagine it is like a jug of water that you are lifting and pouring.

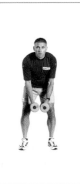

2
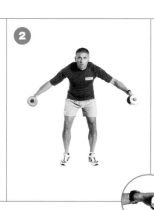

3
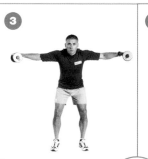

4
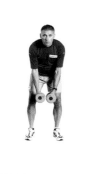

Rotator cuff
Internal and external rotation

You rarely see anybody in the gym working on their rotator cuff muscles. This group of four muscles – the supraspinatus, infraspinatus, subscapularis and teres minor – lie deep within the shoulder area and are critical to the stability of the joint. Most of us don't even know that they're there.

Imagine you are throwing a javelin: you have accelerated quickly, planted your foot and are throwing from the hip. Your arms

and shoulder are also being thrown forwards but since you don't want them to follow the javelin into the air, you have to put the brakes on – and those are your rotator cuff muscles.

They are the muscles that get used by tennis and squash players, swimmers, rugby players grabbing opponents passing at speed. And they are the muscles which prevent your shoulder from getting

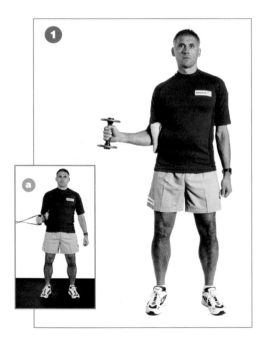

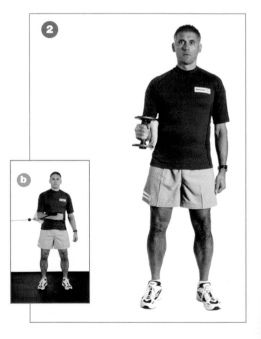

The exercise above is for internal rotation. The start position is with the arm out to your side, then bring it in to a position pointing directly forward from the elbow, as shown on the right. Watch for, and avoid, any tendency to move the weight in and down; keep the movement horizontal.

These simple, subtle exercises are often overlooked, but are crucial to building stronger shoulders.

dislocated. So if you have been building your arms up but have ignored your rotator cuff muscles, it doesn't matter how big your biceps are, they won't stop a dislocation.

This is another subtle exercise: it does not look much, but is incredibly valuable. In both variations – the internal and external rotation – the weight you use can be very very light, as weight is not the issue. It's a good idea to use a folded towel or a small piece of foam between your elbow and hip, to help stop you rotating the hip. The idea is to keep all the body movement to a minimum apart from the movement of the humerus. Maintain a straight vertical stance, with your trunk static and facing forwards. And use the mirror to check your stance, not your hairstyle.

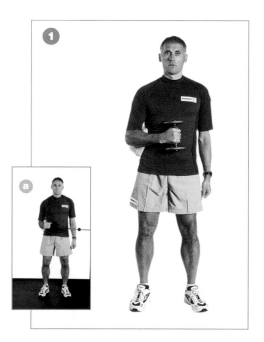

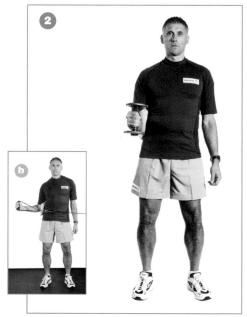

The external rotation starts with your arm across the stomach, before rotating outwards again in a horizontal plane. Don't overextend the arm outwards and keep your body completely static: don't follow the weight, let your shoulder do all the work.

Upright row and shoulder shrugs

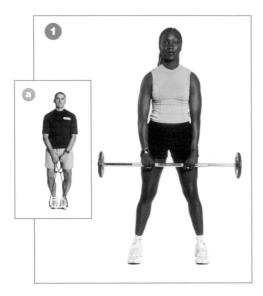

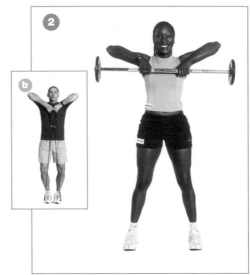

The upright row is a great shoulder and neck exercise, which also incorporates the biceps. The basic exercise brings the barbell up to chest height. In the photos below, I am bringing the bar higher up under my chin, which really brings the traps and the back into use, because you need to shrug your shoulders for that extra bit of lift. Note on this occasion I am using a cable machine set low with a flat bar attachment.

The start position is with your feet slightly wider than shoulder width apart, knees soft, an overhand grip on the bar, hands shoulder width apart. The secret of this exercise is to keep the lift vertical. If you look at the lift side on you should see that the bar brushes up along the stomach throughout the lift – you'll just have to get your beer belly out of the way.

The upright row should also be a controlled exercise when it is forming part of a conditioning programme. Make sure that you lower the bar carefully; don't just let it drop. When doing the reps, counting 'one second up, one second down' will be fine. To increase the intensity of the exercise, you can increase the number of repetitions, and then the weight you're lifting, but keep the speed constant until all the basic conditioning work has been completed. Using heavier weights produces good forearm strength, which you will

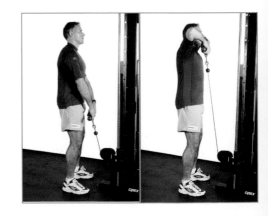

Bernie's tip
The upright row is another exercise where you don't want to get carried away and start lifting too much weight. For most of us, the exercise is for basic conditioning, so lower weights are perfect. You'll notice anyone lifting too much weight on this exercise because they'll lean forward and flick their hip to get the weight moving.

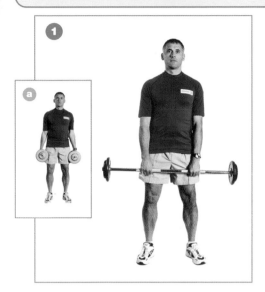

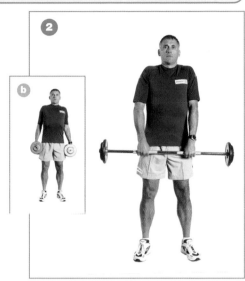

need in the long term to develop your shoulders and upper arms.

As your confidence grows, you can introduce additional variations: a sprinter, for example, may lift the weight very quickly and explosively, then bring the bar down quickly, holding it in the lower position for a long time – and only doing 3 reps per set.

Shoulder shrugs may look deeply dull (and quite frankly I'd agree) but they are extremely good for anyone who is involved in a sport that requires strong shoulder and neck muscles. I've also found this is an exercise I've never had to use with Italian F1 drivers, because they just do it constantly every time they're being interviewed after a race – only kidding, guys!

The shoulder shrug isolates the muscles around the neck. Rugby forwards will use this exercise to create muscle bulk for scrummaging, tackling and rucking. Swimmers and kayakers need it for their

shoulder power. And skiers find it useful to increase the power with which they plant their ski sticks down and push off.

You will be able to lift quite a lot of weight. What will determine how much you can lift, though, is your grip strength rather than your neck muscles. Quite simply you might not be able to lift the weight you want to because your grip gives out. If that's the case, drop the weight back and build your grip strength up gradually.

For the exercise, think about making your shoulders touch your ears: that's the image you should have in your mind. The upright row on the opposite page is all about using the shoulders. This exercise is all shrug. The lifting movement comes from your traps; there should be no arm work at all. When you pick up the barbell or the dumbbells don't use your arms or your back to lift them, use your knees – or take the weights directly off a proper weight rack.

The upper back

- Seated row • Single-arm row • T-bar row
- Lat pull-down • Pull-ups
- Reverse lateral raise • Chest heave

THE UPPER BACK IS ONE OF THE areas for the class-A macho man to work on. Pumping this area up gives him the classic V shape he so badly wants! Fortunately, for the rest of us there's more to this area than a huge pair of lats.

I often come across sportspeople, highly tuned in their own discipline, who struggle in this really neglected area of training. I've had huge rugby players gurning in pain as they lift tiny little weights on the reverse raise (see page 150). They can bench press a small donkey but can't lift a field mouse when it comes to using the deep muscles in the upper back and rear of the shoulders.

Personally, I've recently experienced fatigue in the upper back whilst paddling in my K1. I've often worked the lats and shoulders in the gym but if I neglect the rhomboids and other deeper muscles, that's where it hits me and I feel them fatiguing pretty quickly out on the river. I've also noticed the need for a range of different upper back exercises in sports like climbing, which I now only do from time to time. If you stick with one or two upper back exercises you will get really good at these, but most sports require more than one or two distinct movements. What happens then – in climbing, for instance – is that you recruit the muscle fibres in different ways and from different parts of the muscle because of the ever-changing nature of the moves on a wall; fatigue sets in quickly. It's the law of specificity of training at work and is particularly relevant to this area of the body where most people will only know one or two exercises to use.

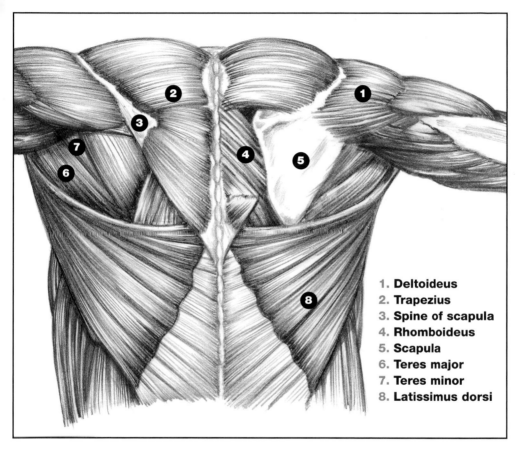

1. **Deltoideus**
2. **Trapezius**
3. **Spine of scapula**
4. **Rhomboideus**
5. **Scapula**
6. **Teres major**
7. **Teres minor**
8. **Latissimus dorsi**

At the other end of the scale, for people who are in the unfortunate position of having to sit at the computer screen all day (and you have my deepest sympathies) the upper back workouts are an important postural activity. Sitting hunched over a keyboard or desk can be complemented brilliantly by the seated row and reverse lateral raises (pages 140 and 150) to straighten you up and sort out those aches and pains you get after a day in the office.

Rowers are very aware of the importance of the back, and of complementing chest exercises with back exercises. The British rowers training at Henley might do some pull-downs specifically to strengthen their backs, and then complement these with bench presses.

In this section we'll look at how to strengthen all the muscles in your back. There is no point having strong shoulders or arms and a weak back – or vice versa – because one set of muscles will have to compensate for the other, and before you know it you'll have an injury.

Seated row

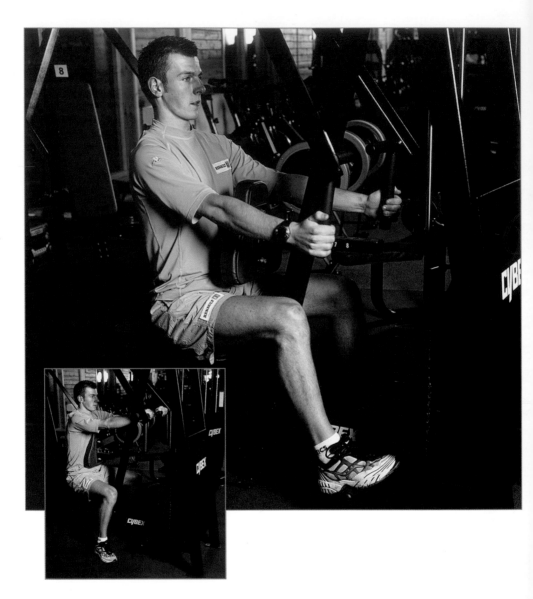

The seated row uses a gym machine to replicate, to a certain extent, the action of expert rowers like Matthew Pinsent and James Cracknell. In the two sets of photos above, the main difference is in the position of the hands. In the two larger photos the hands are vertical in the start position. You will develop good stability in the trunk and the abs to provide the resistance against the weight imposed by the machine, and

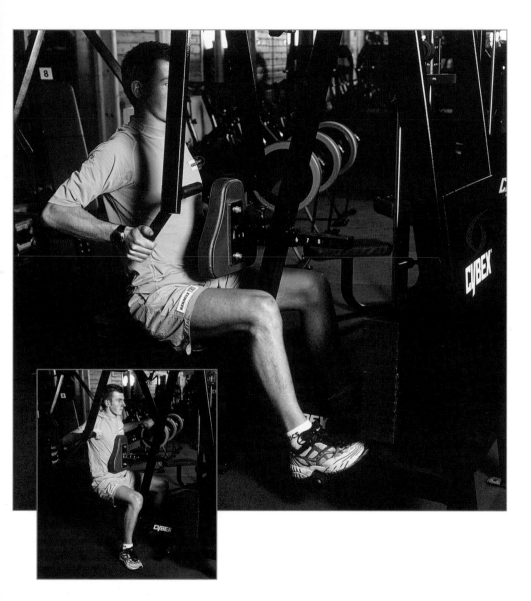

as you draw in your arms the biceps, deltoids and upper back will be worked.

The alternative hand position (in the two inset photos) uses a flat overhand position, with a motion that pulls out and away. This puts less emphasis on the biceps and more on the posterior deltoid and the rhomboids. This version is often – wrongly – neglected, partly because it's easier to lift more with the vertical grip version.

Single-arm row
with dumbbell

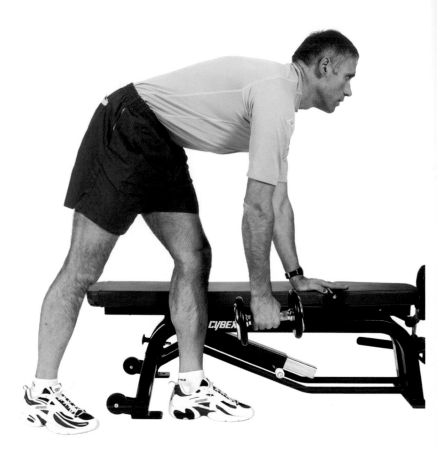

The single-arm row is (as the name suggests) a variation on the seated or T-bar row that allows you to isolate one arm at a time. It works the upper back, biceps and shoulder muscles and is good for building grip strength, as you'll probably be lifting some reasonably big dumbbells after a while.

What you are trying to do is keep a good flat back posture throughout the exercise and avoid rotating the trunk as you lift and lower the weight. If you are doing this, then the chances are you are trying to lift too much weight, so back off a bit and do it right!

The start position is shown in photo 1. Notice the flat back and opposite hand on the bench for balance and support. You can also use an inclined bench to lift the support hand up higher if the bench you are using is too low. When you start lifting heavier weights you may also want to place your knee on the bench for extra support and a more stable base as well.

Pull the weight straight up and really feel your back muscles working by emphasis-

Stay as static as possible; don't rotate your body. To watch out for twisting, use a mirror. Just don't spend too long admiring your hairstyle...

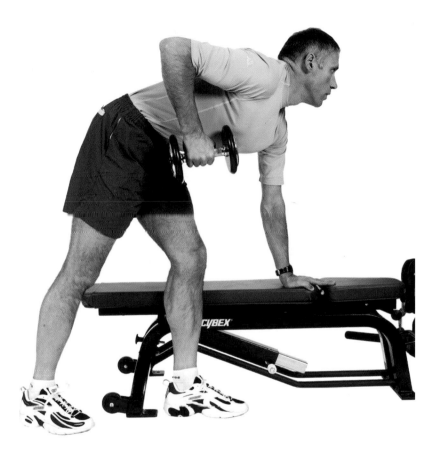

ing the elbow lift at the top of the movement. Don't let the weight drop from the top position either. Lower in a controlled way as this works the muscles eccentrically (as they lengthen) and will stop you damaging your delicate shoulder muscles with a sudden braking movement when your arm ends up straight at the bottom of the exercise. Lastly, be careful when putting the weight down after a set and don't drop it aggressively – it's very close to your foot so I don't think I need to say any more...

Bernie's tip
Try not to go overboard with the weight. You'll only end up rotating your torso and not isolating the right muscles.

T-bar row

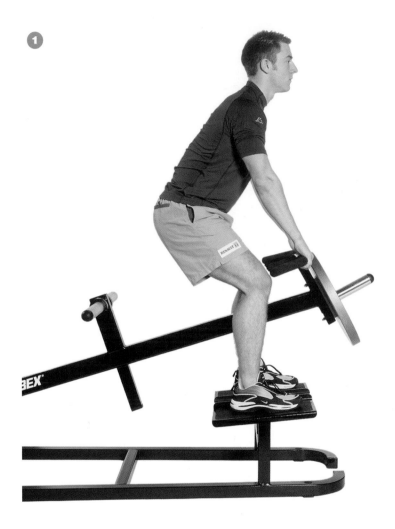

The machine used for the T-bar row is usually brought into operation as part of a specialised strength training programme, but it can also be used for all-round conditioning training. Using this piece of equipment does require a very high level of static strength, so you should not even try to attempt it unless you already have some training under your belt.

Make sure you have a good base, setting the feet shoulder width apart, and squatting down as though you were about to attempt a deadlift, with a flat back. Use your arms and legs to lift the T-bar to the start position – just maintaining this position will be working your back, hips and quads statically (as they will be throughout the entire session). Without altering your position, and keeping your back flat, breathe in hard while

This is no relation to the T-bone steak, even though most people doing it look like they've just eaten eight steaks for breakfast.

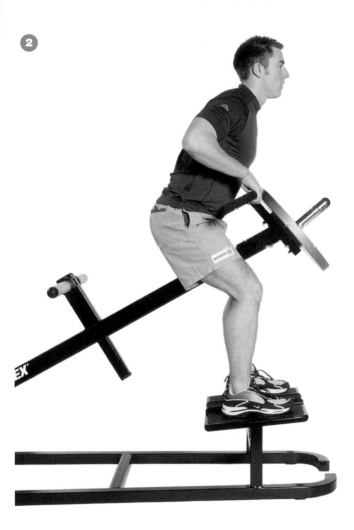

bringing the T-bar up to your trunk, and then lower it under control while returning the bar to the start position. As with all these weights, don't let it go too quickly, as the effects of gravity could have a serious effect on the location of your arm sockets...

I really like this exercise for sports like rowing and rugby. The combination of static and dynamic it requires has huge benefits for total body conditioning and you'll certainly know you've had a good workout when you use this machine; if you do not have access to one, you can simulate the exercise by standing on two boxes and lifting a barbell with only the one weight attached (we've just received an urgent message from the stating-the-bleeding-obvious department: lift the end with the weight on it!).

Lat pull-down

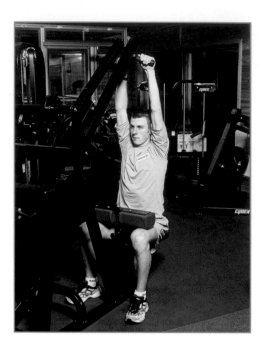 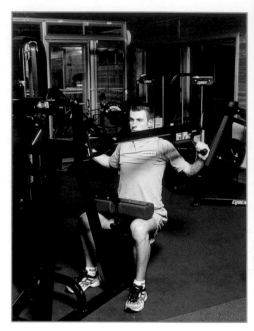

This is a popular exercise, but one that is often performed incorrectly. Have a look next time you're in the gym; you'll see someone loading big weights on the machine (and if you don't see them, you'll soon hear them, because there'll be plenty of grunting and groaning). The great give-away is that the guys who overload this machine will rise up with the weights and then let their own body weight do all the work. This is completely counter-productive – it just proves they weigh too much!

You should be sitting comfortably and solidly, and then bring the weight down to the start position, which is just below your chin at the top of your chest. As you let the bar rise, don't just release it without any control, as you'll be in danger of pulling your arms out of their sockets.

There are a number of variations on the basic exercise: for example, you can turn your hands in and use more of your biceps in the narrower plane.

This is a great exercise for building up to the full pull-up, especially if you don't have access to an assisted pull-up machine. It can be performed on the machine or with cables, kneeling or seated – and is a particularly good exercise for working the lats and bringing the traps into use gradually. Sit or kneel in front of the cables, and with elbows slightly bent, and hands parallel to the floor, pull down until the bar is near your midriff.

A different technique is to sit back subtly and pull the bar to your chest which will bring your shoulders into play much more.

Not so much a pull-down as how do I get down?

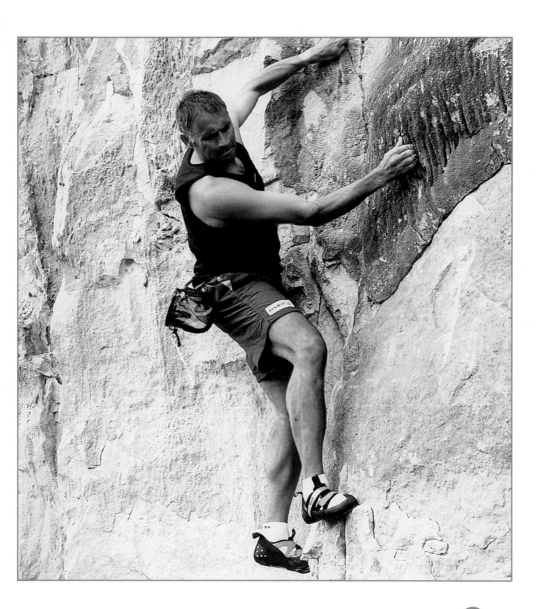

Bernie's tip
I often see people in the gym pulling the bar down behind the neck, but this can be dangerous if you lose control of the movement and catch the back of your head as the bar is jerked upwards. In any case you'll probably need to arch your back to accommodate the movement which is both uncomfortable and unnecessary.

Pull-ups
Assisted and unassisted

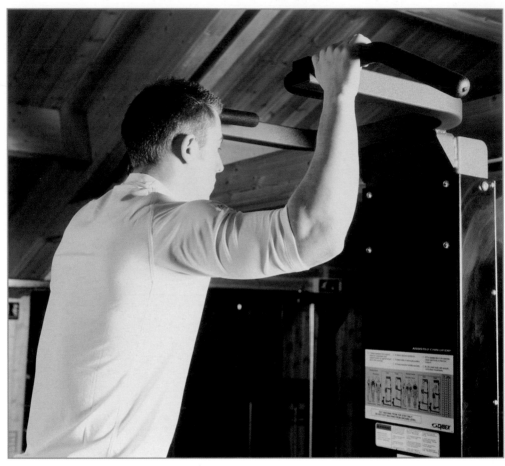

The lat pull-down on the previous two pages is the stepping stone to the full pull-up. Years ago, the pull-up was one of the staples of gym exercise – I remember it well from Marine days ('Let's get Shrosbree on the pull-ups and dips'), but with changing lifestyles and a general increase in body weight it has become less common. With access to gym machines, the assisted pull-up is a superb exercise, since it allows you to control the movement and to use any percentage of your body weight – this gives you the chance to simulate the unassisted pull-up and to move towards the full pull-up safely and progressively. It is also an excellent all-round exercise since the choice of grip works different muscle groups: the underarm grip works your biceps, the overarm your shoulder muscles, likewise a narrower grip will also bring the biceps more into play; a wider grip works the lats and shoulders harder, and for most of us is the harder variation.

I hear a lot of people brag about knocking out sets of 20 or 30 pull-ups, but I'm always sceptical of the quality of their exercise. With this machine 30 good quality pull-ups are possible.

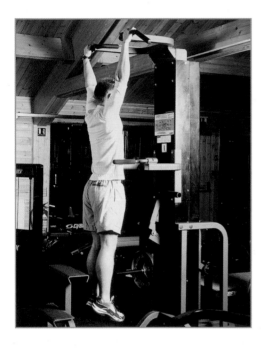

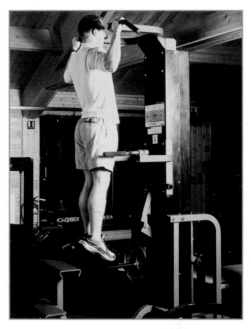

The machine is also the only piece of kit in the gym where the more weight you use, the more it helps you. Start off by entering approximately 80% of your body weight and build from there.

Bernie's tip
On this exercise, go for higher reps with more assistance rather than going for extreme overload to keep the risk of injury down.

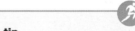

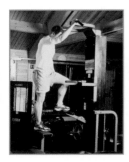

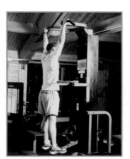

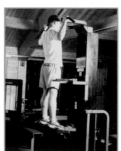

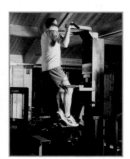

Reverse lateral raise
with dumbbells and cables

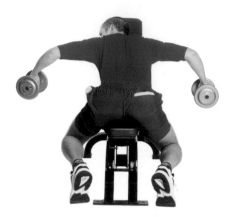

This is an exercise that I don't see people doing very often, and that's a shame, because it really helps work the upper back. Seat yourself face-down on an incline bench, making sure you are comfortable, with your head turned to one side. Pick up the dumbbells and move to the start position which is with straight arms and the weights touching in front of you. Now lift them with bent elbows as if you are trying to touch your elbows behind your back and then – most importantly – squeeze with your shoulder blades. Don't just shrug your shoulders. The way I like to describe it is to imagine you are taking your hands out of your pockets – that's the movement your arms should make. The squeeze is the key: if the weights are too heavy and you can't do the squeeze, then all you are doing is a shoulder raise. Imagine someone has put their finger between your shoulder blades and try to touch that finger.

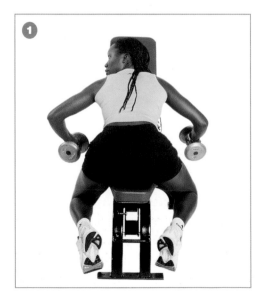

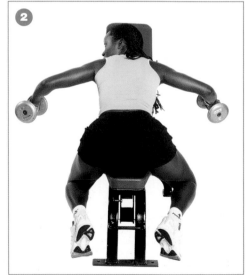

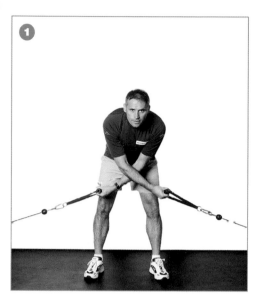

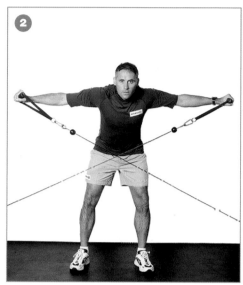

Using the cables: this is my star back exercise. It works almost all the same muscles as the reverse lateral raise, but with smoother resistance because of the effect of the pulleys – and it brings together the static position of the T-bar row on pages 144–145 and the reverse lateral raise. Believe me, you'll get hooked on this exercise. If you have a spare 15 minutes in the gym, this will work out your shoulders *and* your back. The set-up is simple: set the cables up with the pulley system down low, and single hand grips. Stand in the dead centre of the machine, take the cable from the right-hand pillar in your left hand and vice versa, stand with your feet shoulder width apart, and soft knees, lean forwards (the more you bend over the better the squeeze). When you get tired you will tend to stand up, which just recreates a lateral raise. Try to resist this temptation. You *will* get tired, because you are working small muscle groups, so hang on in there.

Bernie's tip
The cables exercise is one of my favourites, but it can be disappointing how little weight you can shift. That's why it's a good one to use with macho rugby players because it helps bring their egos down to size!

Chest heave

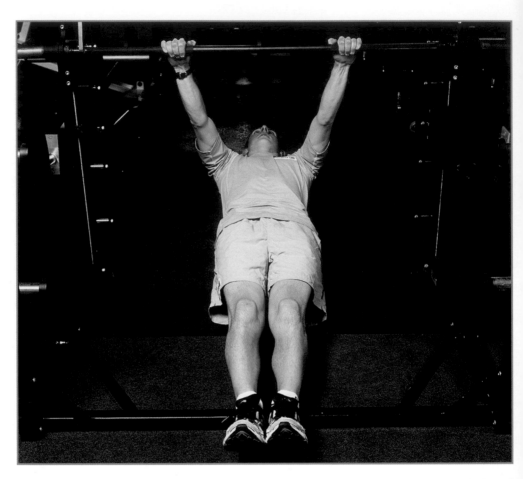

This is another combination exercise and very demanding physically; one that is a high-intensity arm exercise, which also involves your shoulders and back. It will also develop excellent grip strength.

You can use a bench press bar in the gym, or a Smith machine bar (the safest option – though I have been known to use the rails round the edge of a rugby pitch). The bar you use should initially be at hip or waist height. Any higher and the exercise becomes too easy; the lower the bar the more difficult it gets. Lie or sit underneath the bar, grip it and then walk your feet out until you are resting on your heels. Keep your body straight so that there is a rigid link from your shoulders to your heels; you will need good core strength just to hang there. In fact, just hanging there is a good isometric exercise because it is so demanding on your shoulders and your grip, with the loading of virtually your entire body weight.

Then you pull your chin up to the level of the bar, and come back down again.

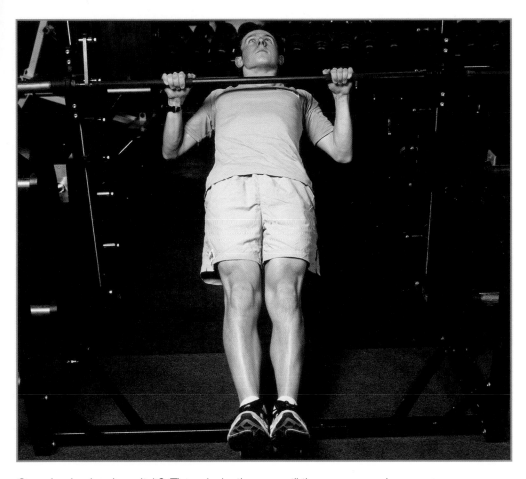

Sounds simple, doesn't it? The grip in the photos is an overhand grip, which works the deltoids. If you want to work your biceps, or if you have weak shoulders, you should swap to an underhand grip.

Climbers develop the kind of strength needed for this because they spend so much time in an overhang position. While a normal, fit person can probably manage 10 chest heaves, a regular climber will do 10 reps, take one arm off, hang by the other, and shake the free arms to get the blood going. Then repeat until the cows come home.

I was once asked by Bournemouth Rugby Club to train the players. They didn't have any equipment so I improvised with the barrier that ran round the edge of the pitch: perfect for chest heaves. I let these burly prop forwards and flankers heave away, told them to do 10 heaves while I went for a coffee, and that if they fell off they'd have to do 10 more. It seemed to wind them up nicely. They had a special name for this exercise. They called it 'the bastard'.

The chest

- **Press-ups** • **Chest press** • **Flys**
- **Cable crossovers**

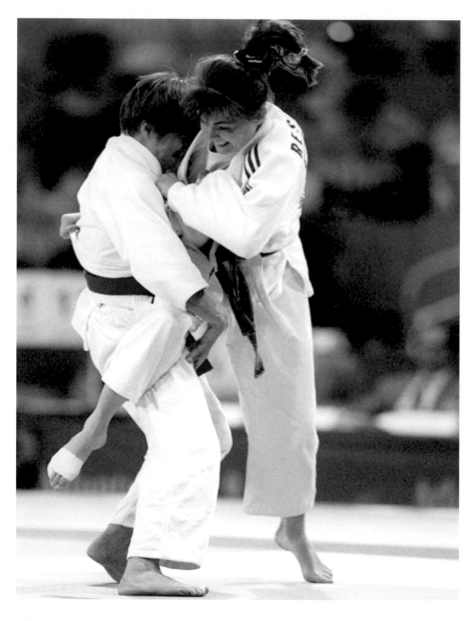

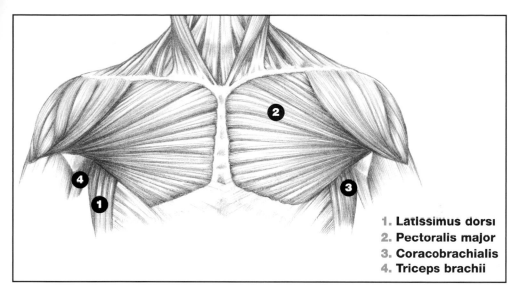

1. **Latissimus dorsı**
2. **Pectoralis major**
3. **Coracobrachialis**
4. **Triceps brachii**

THE MUSCLES OF THE CHEST represent a huge ego zone for guys. Men always seem to be obsessed with building up their pecs – you can even buy a new set down at the surgery so I'm told! The problem with the mentality of focusing – almost to the exclusion of everything else – on the bench press in the gym is that your body develops an imbalance. It's all very well joining the 100 Kilo Club if you want to, but first have a look at the body shape that it creates: rounded shoulders and all the elegant posture of a gorilla. I prefer to treat the chest as another, not the only, important muscle group in the body.

The chest is involved in any pushing and pulling motion. Push something away and the chest and triceps extend the arm. Pull your arm across the body and the chest is doing all the work. It's a large muscle group that gets used on a daily basis – and in a sporting context is critical for any contact sport, and sports involving the arms and shoulders.

Just as it's not a great idea to concentrate too much on building up your chest muscles and ignoring, say, your back, likewise it's not much use having strong arms and a weak chest; otherwise you won't be able to push the arms away.

This muscle group is also an area of concern for women, who are worried that if they spend time working their chest area, it will create an unsightly level of muscle development. The reality is that you would have to work exceptionally hard to see any effect, and in any case chest exercises do not affect the breasts, since they are simply masses of fatty tissue that just rest on the pectoral muscles (I don't think I'll pursue a career as a writer of erotic fiction!).

Press-ups
including box press-up

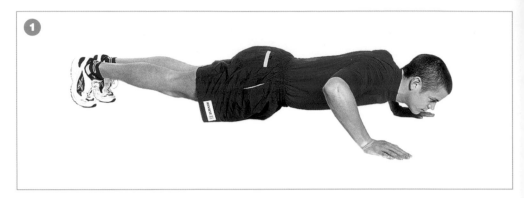

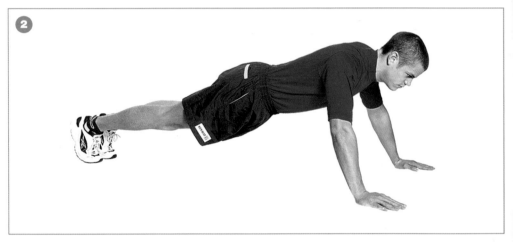

One of the all-time classics – and one of my personal favourites. It's worth getting the press-up right for maximum benefit. No showboating, gents!

This is one of the exercises that everybody knows – and lots of people probably have the wrong impression of. They've seen too many movies where squaddies have been ordered by the drill sergeant to get down and pump out 50 press-ups. The press-up should not be seen as a punishment, nor as a chance to show off.

Like all classic exercises it has become popular because it does the job – in this case, a combined workout of the upper body and the trunk – efficiently and effectively.

A great feature of the press-up is that it can be broken down into degrees of difficulty, so that everyone can tackle the exercise at their own level, from the box press-up through to the full press-up.

Box press-up (photos 3 and 4): this is the one to start with, especially if you

You'll need good core strength to do these. If you're having to stick your bum in the air or you're sagging in the middle, sort out your core strength first.

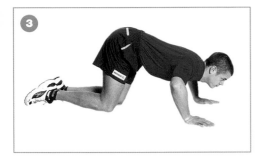

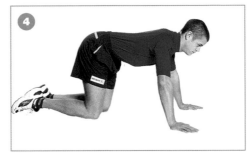

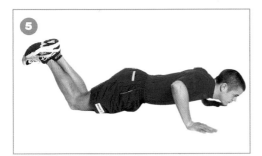

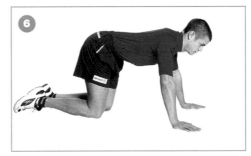

know you have a weak upper body or if you haven't been doing much exercise for a while. Kneel down, making sure that the angle between your legs and backside is 90 degrees. Get your weight over your shoulders, rather than sitting back, and bend your arms down as far as comfortable before pressing through. Always breathe out on the way up (on the exertion).

The three-quarter press-ups (photos 5 and 6): if you are struggling with full press-ups but find box press-ups too easy, try this variation. Start on your knees, push your hips forward and walk your hands forward. Your back and hips should be good and straight, and your head looking straight down. Now drop down until you are the height of a fist only from the

ground. Your hands should be shoulder width apart – they can go further out if necessary to get your body lower at the bottom of the exercise, but don't lock your arms out.

Full press-up (photos 1 and 2): for these you will need good core strength to support your body's structure. If your body starts to judder or sag, then it's telling you that you need to do some more work on your core area (see pages 104–113).

Bernie's tip
There are many variations on the press-up: you can take it slow, or hold the position at the bottom of the exercise to work the muscles statically (something cyclists do). Swimmers often use a plyometric version, pushing off into the air between press-ups and clapping their hands.

Chest press
and incline bench press

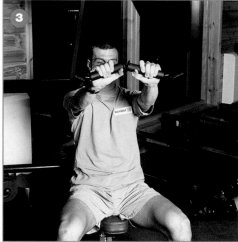

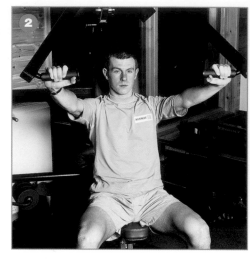

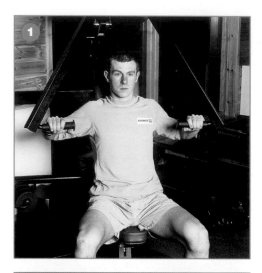

Bernie's tip
Before getting on any weight-stack machine check that the weight load key is set to zero. It's an easy and stupid way to get injured if you don't check first, have no idea what weight is on the machine and suddenly find you're either trying to lift a massive weight that isn't budging, or no weight at all.

The main chest exercise we all know is the bench press. For an in-depth look at this see pages 122–123. The chest press is the machine equivalent of the bench press, just as the pec deck is the machine version of the flys (see pages 160–161).

Before you do anything, make sure that the set-up of the machine is correct: check the seat height, make sure that the handles are across your chest at nipple height. Adjust the width of the hand grips so that they are just outside your shoulder width. Sit back into the seat. As you carry out the exercise don't arch your back, and breathe out on the exertion. If you can hear the weight stacks clanking then either your mechanical set-up is wrong or you're trying to lift too much weight.

If you move from the chest press to free weight bench presses you are suddenly having to provide all the stability. So drop the amount of weight you're lifting to begin with and then increase it as your ability to control the bar and the weights improves.

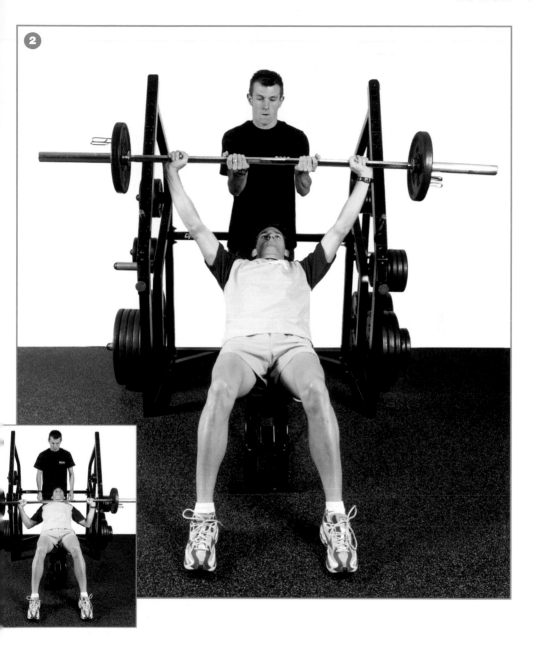

The incline bench press (above) is a variation of the bench press (see pages 122–123). Firstly set the bench at between 45 and 60 degrees. Using an overhand grip, inhale and lower the bar to your upper chest at the base of the neck. Now press the bar up until your arms are straight, exhaling as you complete the movement.

This variation works the upper pectorals and requires more work by the stability muscles in the shoulder.

The exercise should always be performed with a spotter as returning the bar to the rack can become difficult.

Flys
Incline bench fly

1

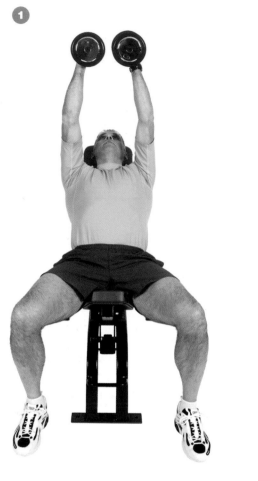

2

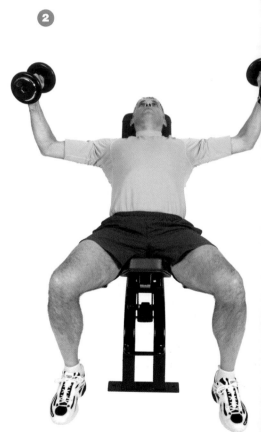

Bernie's tip
Most injuries on flys happen when you overestimate the weight that you can safely lift. This happens because you can lift the weights into position close to the body, but as you pivot them out to the wide position, gravity takes over assisted by a huge lever (your whole arm) and the load goes straight through the delicate shoulder.

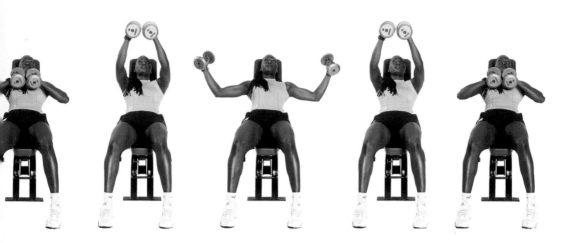

The fly is another one of my favourite exercises: an excellent all-round chest and shoulder workout, and a good element in any strength training programme. But a word of caution upfront. You need to be very, very careful with this exercise; do not lock your arms out straight, because if the load of the weight is too great you are quite likely to do some serious damage to your shoulders, even if your chest and your arms are strong. And if you are working with heavy weights and start to fatigue you can cause shoulder problems. So the message is: take it gently.

The fly can be performed on a flat or inclined bench. The greater the incline, the higher up the pectoral muscles you will be targeting. Whatever the angle, lie with your back on the bench with your feet flat on the floor for support. Start with the weights balanced on your chest, knuckles facing upwards and thumbs towards your chin. Lift the weights slowly in a controlled way to the position shown in photo 1 and then pivoting your arms about the shoulder joint

lower the weights into the position shown in photo 2. Now pivot the arms about the shoulder joint again by contracting your pecs to return to position 1. Note that this is different from a bench press type of action with the emphasis on the weights moving in an arcing motion – not being pressed straight out. From there lower steadily back to photo 2 and repeat. Remember your breathing! For this exercise breathe in as you lower the weights to position 2 and out as you complete the lift in position 1.

At the end of the exercise, bring the weights to your chest and then – in a controlled way – lower them down to the sides. When you are setting up the height of the bench make sure that it is low enough so that your hands can reach the floor. You don't want to get to the end of an excellent set of reps and then find you can't put the weights down on the floor, which means you are either going to drop them or risk a shoulder tear. As always, a minute or two of preparation before going into the exercise will pay dividends.

Cable crossovers

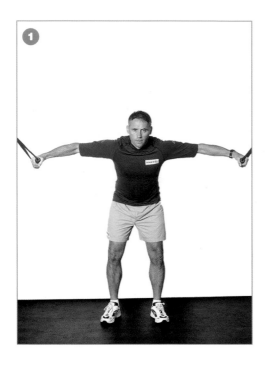

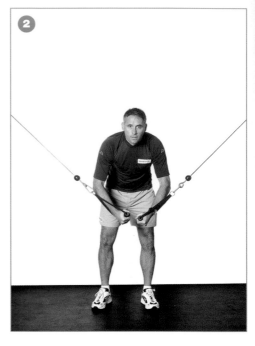

I love the cable rig: it's a really multifunctional piece of kit. And this exercise works particularly well on it. It is a fly but you are standing up and working statically in the trunk as well as working the chest muscles, so it is another example of the kind of combination exercise that I tend to favour for general conditioning. Because of that, you will find it gives you more general exercise than the pure fly, working out your lower back and quads as well.

Once again, take care with the initial set-up, otherwise when you release the position you can end up almost getting crucified! Make sure that the two weight stacks are equally loaded and that you have the same grips on each cable. Stand in the exact middle of the rig – symmetry is important in this exercise.

Your arms are working independently, and you will naturally have a dominant side, so work to the weaker of the two rather than the stronger. Stand with your feet shoulder width apart and with soft knees. Tilt your hips slightly forwards, stomach in, elbows high (photo 1) and then bring the

Bernie's tip
Try not to bend over too much using the lower back excessively – if you're doing this you've probably got too much weight on – drop the loading and do it properly!

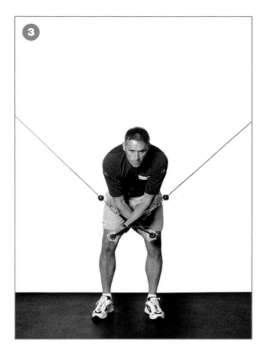

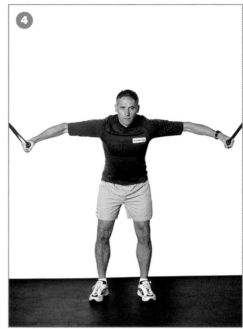

two arms into the centre with your elbows slightly bent and keeping your head high, looking forwards (photo 2).

Don't use your biceps; pull your arms as a single unit and then cross them over (photo 3) for the extra squeeze that will work the pecs. It doesn't really matter which arm is in front of the other, though most people use their dominant arm in front since it requires a little more work.

On the recovery (photo 4) avoid clunking the weights; just kiss the weights back into position and then move seamlessly into the next rep. This exercise requires smooth continuous reps – don't plop the weights back and have a five-minute rest between each lift.

This is just one of a huge variety of exercises you can perform on the cable machine – be inventive. When you get really good at the core balance on the exercise ball, try this exercise by sitting on a ball instead of the normal standing position. Hold your posture upright as you perform the exercise and feel your abs and lower back working really hard to stabilise your core. Start with your feet out at about shoulder width for maximum support and gradually move them in together as your strength increases. Alternatively try kneeling on the ball; both variations are really hard but add a new dimension of core stability work to the exercise. More core exercises are on pages 104–113.

The arms

- Biceps curl • Concentration curl
- Triceps extension and kickback
- Machine and bench dips

WHEN I WAS A MARINE, I NEVER HAD those massive, pumped-up arms that you see on the guys working flat out in the gym, so in typical military fashion the PTIs always took great delight in announcing, 'OK, let's get Shrosbree doing dips and pull-ups.'

The arms are an area of the body where there is a lot of pressure to have the biggest muscles, that whole macho thing about building up your 'big guns'. There's nothing wrong with that particularly, but if

you concentrate too much on your arm muscles you may well find that your whole body is getting out of balance.

Work on your arms by all means, but ensure at the same time that all the supporting muscles are equally well-conditioned. If you're a yachtsman, for example, large biceps are great for the strength you need to sheet in, but if you've neglected your forearms you simply won't have the grip strength to

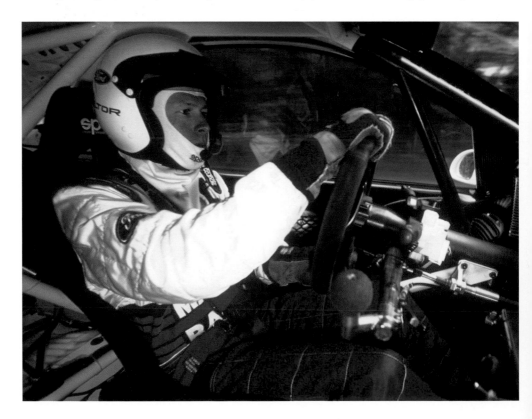

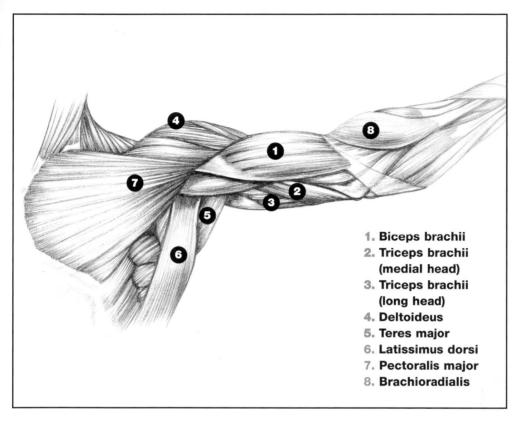

1. **Biceps brachii**
2. **Triceps brachii (medial head)**
3. **Triceps brachii (long head)**
4. **Deltoideus**
5. **Teres major**
6. **Latissimus dorsi**
7. **Pectoralis major**
8. **Brachioradialis**

hold the ropes after a while. Apart from those lovely big muscles not being quite as effective if they're the only ones you've been building up, you also run the risk of incurring injuries through overuse and imbalance.

Women usually have a different area of concern, worrying that working on the arms will create an unflattering, bulky look, which is of course a complete myth. Having well-conditioned arm muscles doesn't mean you have to look like the Incredible Hulk, as long as you set yourself sensible goals and work on developing those muscles gradually; as with the chest,

building muscle mass is very difficult and shouldn't concern 99% of gym users.

There are three aspects of working the arm (or any other) muscles: conditioning, strength and power training. Of these three, the most important is the conditioning phase, using high repetitions and low weights/resistance. This can help anybody in simple, daily activities – like lifting boxes up into the attic or hoicking one of your kids up into the air – as well as for those sports where well-conditioned arms are a bonus, if not a must (kayaking, rowing, rugby and netball, for example). All of the exercises in this section will help.

Biceps exercises 1
Biceps curl with barbell, dumbbell and cables

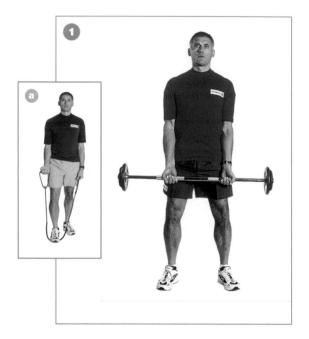

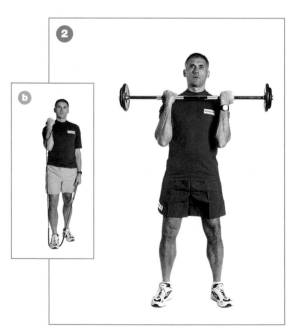

The biceps curl does what it says on the tin. By curling your biceps muscle you are working it through all its actions: bending the arm (technically called 'flexion'), extending the arm ('extension'), and turning your palm to the front ('supination').

You can work with either dumbbells or a barbell. Working with the barbell allows you to have greater control over the action, and gives you more balance between your two arms. You may find – as many people do – that you have a dominant arm; you should aim to achieve an equal balance. However, if you are doing biceps curls for the first time and don't feel particularly confident, or if you suffer from lower back problems, start out with the dumbbells.

The key to this exercise is keeping a strong base. If your base is not stable – and especially if you are trying to lift heavier loads than your body can cope with – you may end up straining your lower back.

If you are working with the barbell (left), find a good surface, so that your base is solid. Stand with your feet shoulder width apart, back straight, and use an underhand grip on the bar; your hands should be just over shoulder width apart. Breathe in as you curl the arms upwards, then breathe out as you bring the arms back down. In strength work, some people will subtly lift their heels to avoid falling backwards – this just puts excess stress on the back region. What you can do is stand with your back against a wall which will keep your back straight, but avoids undue stress and the danger of twisting with the weight. Also remember to keep your knees 'soft' and not lock them out.

Overdo this one, or do it without a full ROM, and you'll get shortened muscles like the guys who look as if they've been carrying rolls of lino under their arms all day.

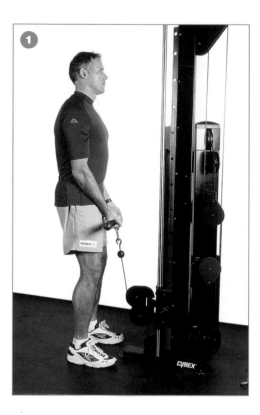

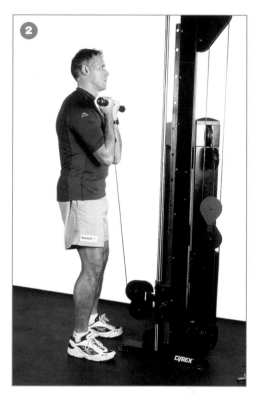

Remember that each of us is an individual and we all have different lever lengths. So work within your capabilities and don't get fazed by what other people are lifting, otherwise you might find that minor injuries start to happen.

You can also use a bungee cord to replicate the action of the curls (as shown in pictures a and b on the left), or use a cables machine as above. For this, set the pulley as low as possible. Bend the knees, raise the bar using an underhand grip to a comfortable position about mid-thigh. Then complete the action as if you were using a barbell. Keep the muscle under tension as you lower the weights to the start position, i.e. don't lock out your arms at the bottom or rest when the weights are stacked.

Bernie's tip
The word 'biceps' means 'two-headed' – there is a short and long head in the muscle. To work these separately, you can adjust your grip on the barbell. Bring the hands closer together to work the long head, move them wider apart to work the short head.

Biceps exercises 2

Concentration curl, hammer curl and reverse curl

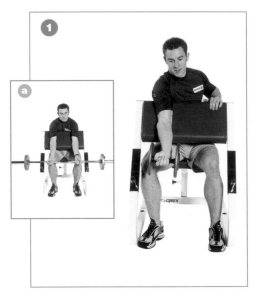

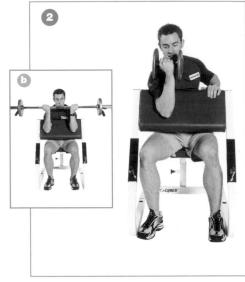

The preacher curl does much the same as the biceps curl, but by using the perch (or angled bench) to support the back of your arms, you are isolating the biceps quite precisely. As before, breathe in as you curl up, out on completing the movement. Warm up well before trying this exercise as it puts considerable stress on the muscles when your arms are extended.

We are – as with all these arm exercises – trying to minimise any movement of the body except in the arms, so that the muscles we want to isolate are doing all the work.

To keep a balance between the two arms, do one set of reps with one arm and then swap to the other for the next set; this will help the muscle to recover between sets. If you are a tennis player or rower, you may find that you are one-sided, so use alternating reps to balance your arms. When James Cracknell was asked to swap sides in the boat, he needed to readjust his balance – we call it 'neuromuscular re-education' in the trade if you want to impress your training partner.

The hammer curl is a variation to target the brachioradialis and other forearm muscles. It takes its name from the grip you would naturally use to lift a hammer. You should use a full range of motion, completing the lift when the dumbbell touches the shoulder.

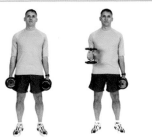

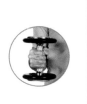

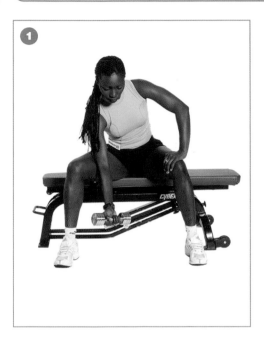

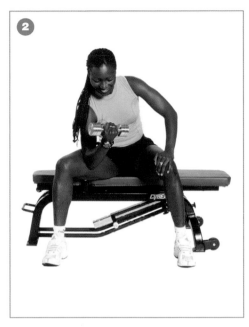

The concentration curl is another pure biceps exercise but this time you will be isolating the muscle by resting your elbow on your leg. This is the exercise that will give you those big guns, if you want them.

Sit on a bench, feet firmly on the floor, use an underhand grip on the dumbbell, and rest your elbow on the inside of your thigh.

Then lift your arm and turn your palm to face up; curl the arm and then return it to the start position. As you raise the weight breathe in, then out on the way down. You can either repeat that with the same arm, or alternate between both arms.

To lift significantly heavier loads (for sports like rugby, javelin, shot put and, obviously, weightlifting), you may need help to get over the pivot point on both these exercises. Don't be brave, use a 'cheat'; get someone to assist you in moving the weight over the fulcrum.

The curl with reverse grip. This variation targets the extensors of the wrist and is excellent for improving forearm strength. It uses the brachioradialis to a greater extent than the biceps.

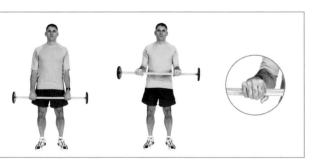

Triceps exercises 1
Triceps extension and kickback

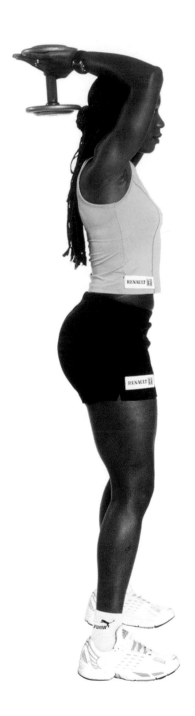

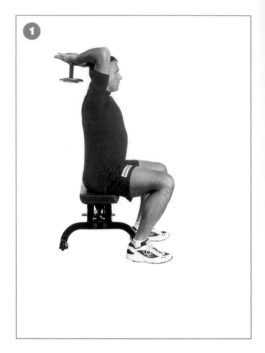

1

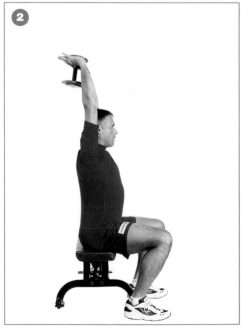

2

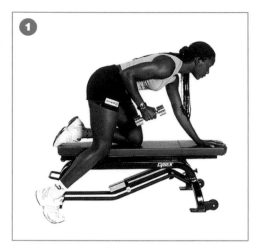

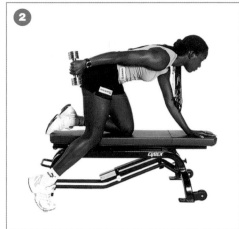

After the biceps these next exercises concentrate on the triceps muscle, the muscle at the back of your upper arm that straightens your elbow. Tricep means 'three-headed' – which is obvious once you think about it – and the exercises here will work all three heads. Raising and stretching the triceps is very good for sports like cross-country skiing (for the push-off), swimming (in the last part of a stroke) and any sports that involve throwing or pushing.

When you are in a deep armchair watching the Six Nations, and you have to push yourself up and out of the chair to get another beer, that's the triceps muscle you're using. If you're out on the rugby field, you'll be using the same muscles every time you push a tackler away.

For the triceps extension (left), you can stand or sit, but either way make sure your posture is good and firm, that your back is not arched and that your base support is solid. Hold the dumbbell behind your neck using both your hands, with the palms upwards. From the starting position – with the dumbbell behind your head – breathe in and then extend your arms above your head in a straight line, and concentrate on keeping your back straight too. This is one of the rare exercises where you can lock out your arms at the top of the movement.

The triceps kickback uses the bench for support. Softly flex the knees, bend forward at the waist, and start the exercise with your arm bent at an angle of 90 degrees. Then breathe in as you straighten your arm backwards, keeping your upper arm pressed against your side; breathe out as you return to the start position.

The key to the triceps kickback is using a light weight; you are trying to condition the muscle, but not increase bulk.

Bernie's tip
As well as being good preparation for skiing, the triceps kickback is great for tennis and squash – when you extend your arm at the end of a serve or a cross-court backhand.

Triceps exercises 2
Machine dips and bench dips

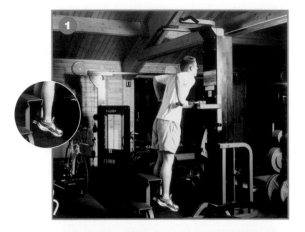

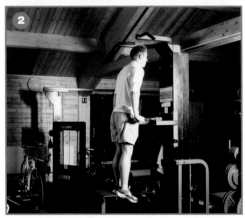

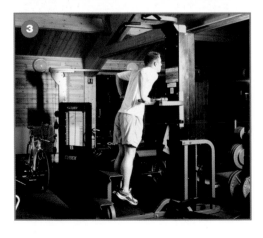

These exercises are a progression from the triceps extension and kickback on the previous two pages. You need to be stonger to do them, so make sure your basic conditioning is in place before attempting either exercise.

This is one of my favourite machines because those of us who are a little weaker in the arms can utilise the counterweight to control the intensity of the exercise.

By which I mean you can increase the weights on the machine which will counteract your own body weight, allowing you to dip below 90 degrees if you want.

When using this machine, range of movement (ROM) is all important. It's no good if you're hardly moving at all. Aim to dip down to a 90-degree bend in the arm. Keeping the body upright will emphasise your arms, if you lean forward the chest comes more into play.

Once the movement is comfortable and you have reached a plateau, you can increase your effective body weight by decreasing the counterweight, having none at all, or even wearing a weight belt.

The bench dips (right) are an exercise you can do either in the gym or at home, and are a valuable component of speed-circuit training. Start off by sitting on the edge of the bench with your heels resting on the box, your knees softly bent. Your hands should be about shoulder width apart, with your hands resting on the edge of the bench as shown in the pictures.

From the start position, lower yourself down, bending at the elbows to approximately 90 degrees, breathing in as you go down and exhaling on the way back up.

I often see guys working on triceps dips, looking like nodding donkeys, which tells me they're not strong enough to do it properly. Get some counterweights on!

When you come back up don't lock your arms out, just bring them to a comfortable straight position, otherwise you will be putting too much pressure on the elbow.

Keep your head still and the core of your body static so that the flexion and extension of your elbows is the only active movement. Then try to establish a good, flowing rhythm; for conditioning work the whole movement down and back up should take around three seconds (for speed training, where the emphasis is on explosive movement, you will be trying to do the movement as quickly as possible).

If you find that you are initially struggling to do, say, 8 or 10 repetitions then consider the option of building up your conditioning by doing the same exercise but with your feet on the floor (lower two pictures) to allow yourself to get used to the exercise. But make sure that the movement is through your arms, and you're not cheating by letting your hips do all the work.

How high should the box be? Essentially the higher the box, the higher the resistance, and the more difficult the exercise and the strain on your triceps. I would suggest starting with a box that is lower than the bench you are using and take it gently. As I'm sure you know by now, I am a believer in taking things gently. Don't overstrain any muscles, but work them with a gradually increasing intensity – otherwise you may pay dearly. These dips may look a little timid at first sight, but, believe me, they are very demanding on your triceps.

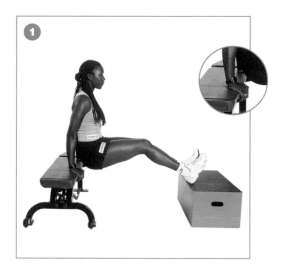

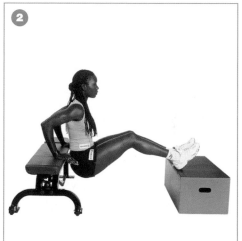

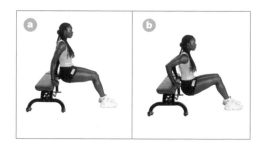

Triceps exercises 3

and combination arm exercises

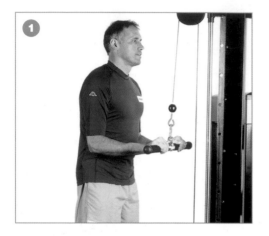

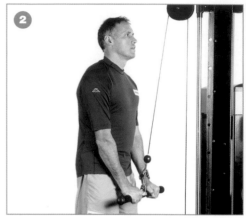

If your gym has a pulley system you can use it to vary your arm exercises. For the triceps, use either a bar or the rope, and set up the pulley system as high as it will go, as shown. Stand upright, either placing both hands on the bar or gripping the rope and keeping your elbows tucked well into your sides throughout the exercise. Push your arms down as far as they will go. If you're using the rope the final movement on the lowest part of the exercise is to subtly twist your hands out and away. Then return the rope or bar to the start position, all the time keeping your elbows tucked in. Do the exercise slowly and with complete control.

A common mistake with this exercise is to use too much weight. Keep it relatively modest. And watch out that you are not leaning out, which will work your back and chest you need to keep yourself well tucked in.

The rope pull exercise on the right is variation which works both the biceps and then the triceps as you pull through. You arm endurance will benefit from this and can be used to enhance your swimming and kayaking.

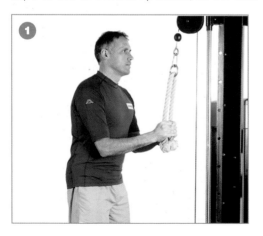

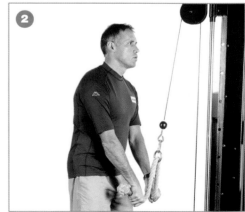

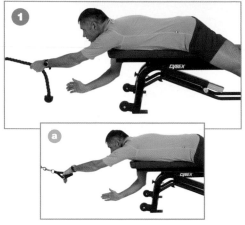

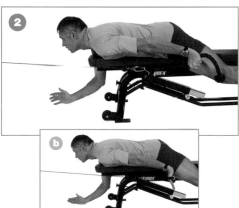

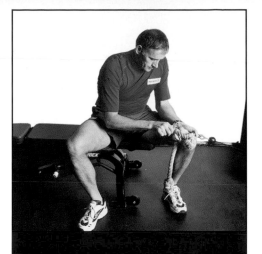

The rope pull is a relatively unconventional kind of exercise, but the kind I love because it gives the whole arm a workout. The initial part of the exercise works your shoulders and biceps, then your triceps, deltoids and finally your lats come into play – an excellent combination exercise. In addition, your grip strength is developed because you are holding onto the rope, so your wrists and forearms will benefit. By doing one exercise you are probably getting more all-round benefit than lots of sets of the individual muscle exercises. Not only will a multi-task exercise like the rope pull benefit a lot of different sports (particularly swimming, rugby and racquet sports like tennis, badminton and squash) but it is an incredibly efficient way of training if you only have 40 minutes in your lunch hour to nip out to the gym.

A few words about the wrist. If you play tennis, badminton, squash or enjoy rowing or kayaking, you'll appreciate the importance of good grip. Here are a couple of exercises designed to build that up. The wrist roll isolates the muscle groups in the wrist and forearm just as the single arm curl or concentration curl does for the biceps. Place your wrist on a raised bench and your free hand on top of your forearm to make sure all the movement is focused in the right areas. Grip the dumbbell with an underhand grip and curl up. This works the topside of the forearm (turn your hand over and curl back to work the complementary muscle). The wrist rotation uses the same principles, but moves the wrist muscles in a different plane. Grip one end of a dumbbell with the shaft upright above your hand, then rotate left and right. You can also work with a gyroscopic weight inside a rigid ball. I've concentrated on grip/wrist strength with rally drivers, where the ability to grip the wheel if the power steering blows is essential, and after hours on a bumpy, unforgiving road that extra percentage of strength can make a few vital seconds of difference.

The trunk and lower back

- Trunk curls • Oblique crunch
- Side bends • Reverse curl
- Hip extensions • Good morning

THE TRUNK, OR MID-SECTION, IS made up of all the muscle groups in the lower back, the obliques and the abdominals, as well as the underlying muscles that act like an inner tube around your whole midriff.

The trunk and lower back is a very important area to concentrate on – and yet it's one that many, if not most, people fail to understand fully. There is always a new batch of fads and techniques which claim to improve your trunk (a few actually do), and a bunch of gadgets like the lumbar supports for car seats. We have become increasingly reliant on creating ways of supporting posture rather than doing anything to get our posture right in the first place. Our lifestyles have become lazy; if our trunks are out of shape, our backs will suffer. Consequently it's not surprising that every year hundreds of thousands of days off work are blamed on a 'bad back' – and not just because it's a convenient excuse.

I've lost count of the times I've heard people tell me, 'I only bent down to pick a pencil off the floor, and my back went.' The truth is that their back hasn't suddenly 'gone'. It will actually have been 'going' for a long time, because their muscles have not been getting the right kind of exercise. As a result, one simple action – lifting a box, maybe just reaching out to take a plate from the back of the dishwasher – was the straw that broke the camel's back. You may

find that you're getting a weak back if your job involves prolonged periods of time sitting at a desk hunched over a computer, or hours driving your car between meetings.

There are as many myths as misconceptions about the trunk. We all know the image of the supposedly superfit guy locking his toes under the bedframe and levering himself up time after time, but that's not what the trunk is all about. Sit-ups alone do not provide the answer. Doing fifty sit-ups makes you good at sit-ups but not much else.

To have a strong trunk you do not have to perform trunk exercises alone. Weightlifters and canoeists may never do a sit-up but they have very strong core strength because of the nature of the sport they perform. After taking up marathon paddling I have found I don't need to do many specific trunk exercises. I get all the workout I need from the static work in the boat, and the twisting motion, with my feet pressed against the footrest and the paddle pressed down against the water is just as good, if not better, than a crunch.

When I was working with firefighters, I used to get them to hold their breathing apparatus above their heads and then lean over by 15 degrees to pass the apparatus along – and the interesting thing was they couldn't hold the position. They had excellent upper body strength but very weak backs and obliques. If you can

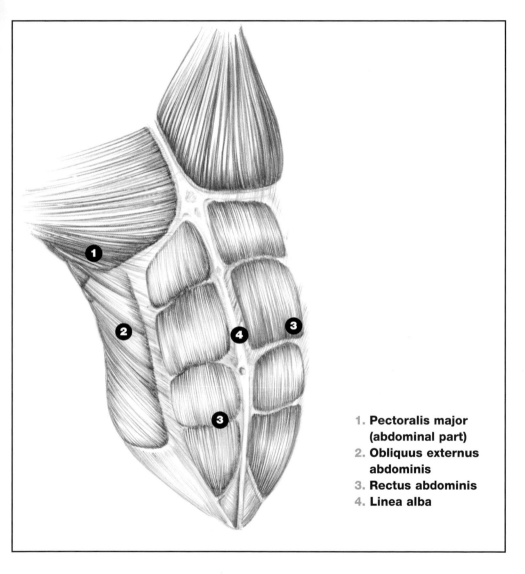

1. **Pectoralis major (abdominal part)**
2. **Obliquus externus abdominis**
3. **Rectus abdominis**
4. **Linea alba**

maintain and improve your core and trunk muscles, your back will be stronger and your rotation better. If you spend some time painting the ceiling or raking leaves you'll see how vulnerable the trunk is, and how quickly the muscles tire.

In this section I have identified some specific trunk and lower back exercises, but remember that all-round core strength and conditioning is just as important (see pages 104–113).

Trunk curls

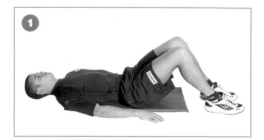

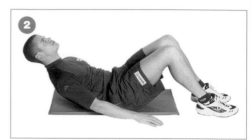

The trunk curl, or the sit-up, is – along with the press-up – one of the exercises that almost everybody has attempted at some point in their life. And like the press-up, it's an exercise that is easy to get wrong.

The basic technique (photos 1 and 2) is to lie down on your back on a good flat, soft surface, preferably a training mat. Your knees should be bent, your feet flat on the floor and shoulder width apart, and your arms flat by your sides with the hands flat on the floor and your head fully back on the floor.

Then fix a point on the ceiling above you to concentrate on and as you lift your head up blow out – as though you're blowing out the candles on a birthday cake. You'll feel your trunk working hard.

For the correct head position, imagine you've got a tennis ball under your chin (in fact, you can actually do this exercise holding a ball there). Trying a small number of reps until you fatigue will give you a pretty instant guide as to the condition of your abs.

There are a number of levels that you can work through. Start with the basic trunk curl. If you are struggling even to raise your shoulders off the floor, then you may simply need to work on your weight initially. If you feel comfortable doing the basic position, move onto the same movement but increasing the difficulty factor by keeping your arms crossed on your chest (photos 3 and 4) and then touching your ears or temples (photos a and b).

Don't start on these harder versions until you are completely comfortable with the basic exercise.

Variations on the main theme include working with a ball gripped between or on your shins with your lower leg held at 90 degrees (see photos 5 and 6). This will help increase the static stress around your hips – and again, you can increase the difficulty by moving on to the heavier medicine balls. In some specific sports at an extremely advanced level, in boxing or rowing for example, the athletes may place a 20kg weight on their chest and perform the exercise while a trainer holds down their legs, but please note, this should only be done as part of supervised training with a qualified instructor.

Bernie's tip
You don't have to do trunk curls all the time. Mix them up with some kayaking or hiking with a backpack, where your trunk has to support the load. Try to keep your exercise routines varied. Don't ever let yourself get bored.

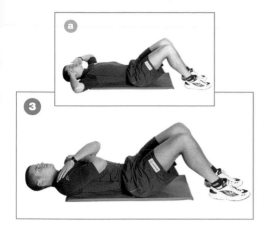

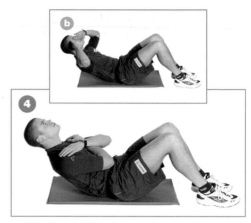

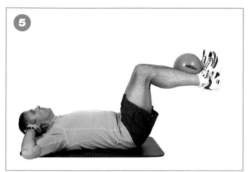

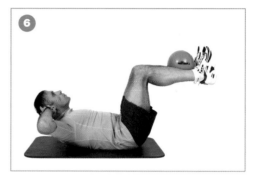

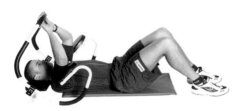

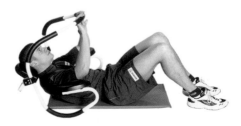

Cradle curls

In the mid-1990s, the trunk curl cradle became extremely popular; you'll find a few of these available at most gyms. There was a whole rash of gizmos which hit the market at about the same time, but this was one of the better ones, because it provides neck support and controls the arcing shape of the motion that you need to do, helping you achieve a good abs exercise.

It is also convenient if you are exercising at home, and doesn't take up acres of space in the living room.

For the starting position, you should crawl underneath the cradle and place the nape of your neck on the pad, bending your legs, with your feet shoulder width apart, and then placing the back of your upper arms against the arm pads.

Advanced variations include:
• crossing your feet in the air
• using a medicine ball

Oblique crunch
and cable crunch with twist

If you want to concentrate specifically on your oblique muscles, the exercises shown on the next few pages will help. The oblique crunch (in the photos below) is a relatively soft version to get you started. Begin with the basic position for a trunk curl (see the previous pages) but place your left arm across your waist and touch your right hand to your right temple. Then you come up as for a trunk curl, but at the top of the lift, turn your trunk towards the left. To work the obliques on your other side simply reverse the process, so that when you come back up you turn to the right.

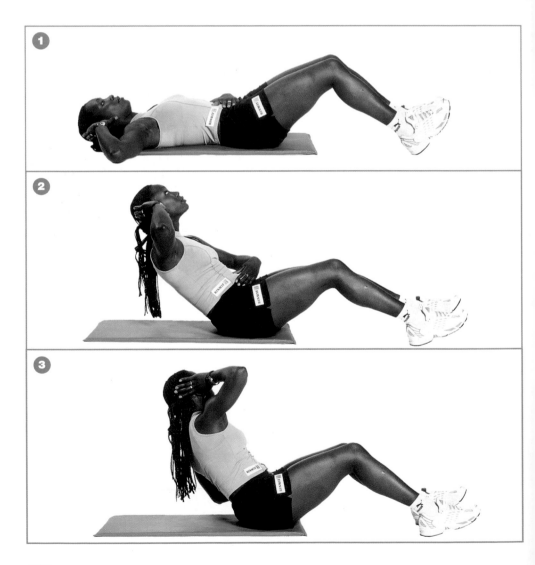

If you want that poser's six-pack, remember that 500 crunches a day won't do it alone. You also need to do some aerobic training to trim down your beer belly and reveal that washboard!

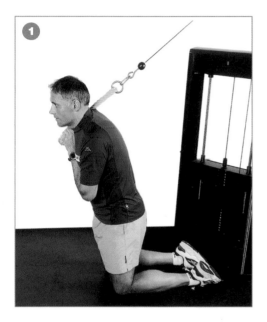

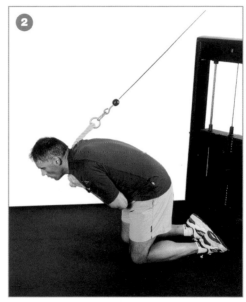

The cable crunch is a more sports-specific variation, because if you think about it there are very few sports where you will be required to perform a crunch while lying on the ground or on your back.

Kneeling, as shown above, and using a cable, replicates more faithfully the kind of position you might be adopting if you are in a kayak, for example. I have found this exercise very useful in building up my lower

back and abs, as well as my obliques.

Kneel on a pad, with the rope coming over one shoulder. Grasp hold of it with both hands (this is an exercise that is good for grip strength too) and then do a forwards crunch. When you feel you have reached the maximum forward movement, drop the shoulder which has the rope on it to get some additional movement and to work those obliques.

Bernie's tip
Be subtle with your crunches and hold good form while you perform them. Think quality not quantity to get results.

Side bend
with variations

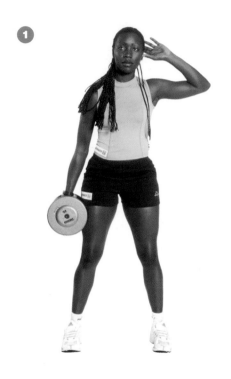

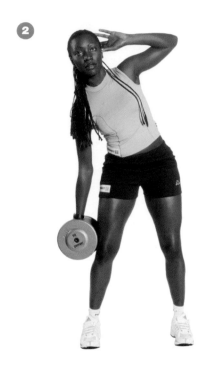

The side bend is a good combination exercise, which targets the obliques, but also works the shoulder muscles. If your obliques need conditioning this is a good exercise to complement any work you are doing on your abs.

The basic exercise with a dumbbell is quite straightforward. Stand with your feet shoulder width apart, soft knees, and one dumbbell held using an overhand grip, the other arm touching your head lightly at the temple for stability.

Then bend to one side and come back up. There should be absolutely minimal rotation or twist, which you can check by looking in the gym mirrors. Slide the weight gently down alongside your leg, rather than leaning over and letting it drop,

keeping the exercise under control all of the time. The end of the bend will be determined by your range of movement, which varies enormously from person to person. Some of us have very good lateral flexion, while others are extremely stiff in that direction.

The side bend can sound (and indeed can be) quite boring; sometimes you feel that you might as well just roller the ceiling and tie a weight to the roller! So you can bring in extra movement by using a medicine ball (see right). This is more taxing and works the shoulders harder because the weight is above shoulder height and adds plenty of resistance – it is a very good exercise for your range of movement and flexibility generally.

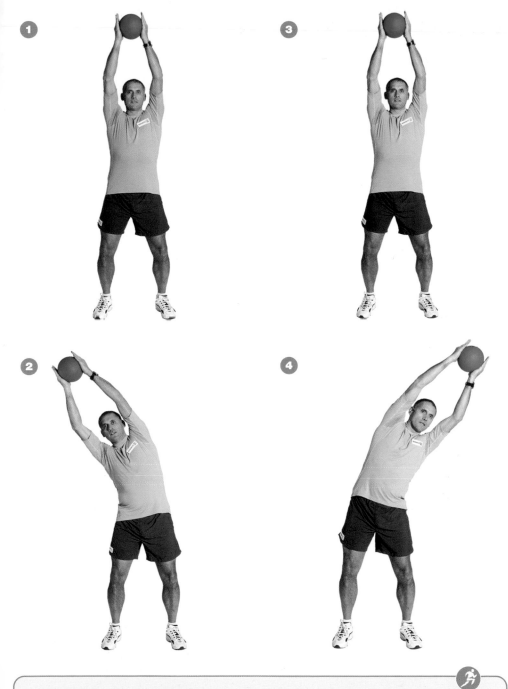

Bernie's tip
Like the calf raise (see pages 196 and 197), the side bend is a subtle exercise because it is not very flashy but it gives a great return. The benefit it can bring to your range of movement, especially using the medicine ball, is great if you want to tone yourself up for sports with lots of turning motion – maybe a return to the village cricket team after a few years off...

Reverse curl
hip flexors and hip extensions

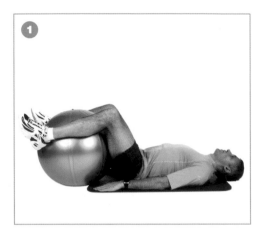

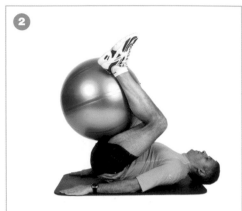

These three exercises work the hip flexors, extensors and abs. The reverse curl is one I use a lot in circuit training because it works so many muscles as well as the hips – and I also find it extremely useful for anybody with lower back problems or poor mobility. Also, you can start at a low intensity and control the difficulty by changing the size of the ball (start with one about 50 or 60cm in diameter). The larger the ball the easier it is to control since the ball limits the range of movement required.

Keep your back flat, your head flat on the ground, your hands three or four inches away from your hips out to the side with the palms flat on the floor. This is so you don't start cheating by putting your hands under your backside!

Try to lift the ball up quickly and lower it down slowly but don't let it rest on the floor at the end of each rep – keep the tension in the muscles by hovering just an inch or so off the deck.

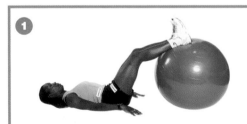

Hip extension: make sure your basic conditioning is good before you try to move on to the hip extension. Unlike the reverse curl, this is a case of the bigger the ball the more difficult the exercise, so start off with a smaller ball.

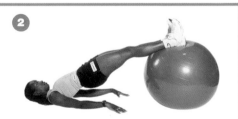

Place your feet on the ball, the top half of your body lying on the floor as if for a reverse curl. Then raise your hips up and off the floor and hold the position statically with your stomach in. Remember to keep breathing!

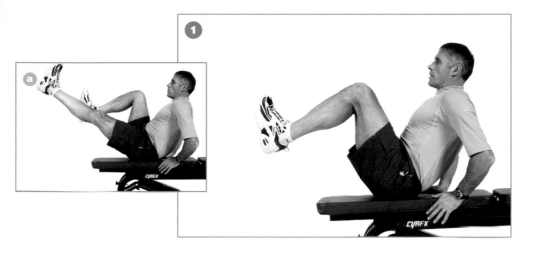

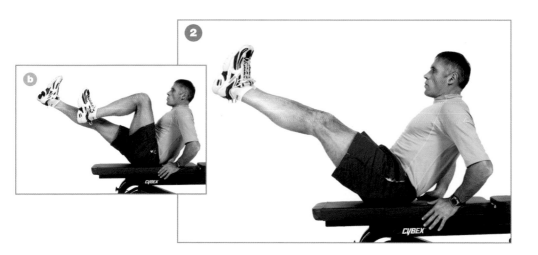

These kickouts are another circuit training favourite of mine, which can either be done with your legs together (as in photos 1 and 2) or alternately as in photos (a and b). Sit on the bench with your hands behind your back, gripping the edge of the bench so that you are well supported. Bend the knees and kick the leg(s) through smoothly but quickly 'see-sawing' at the waist. Keep your heels high (don't point toes) and breathe in rhythm with the exercise. This exercise should be done at a fairly rapid rate so make sure you are well warmed up before taking it on.

Advanced trunk work

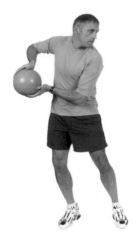

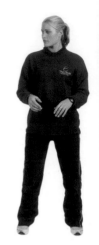

As I travel the world training in gyms and sports clubs with a range of top athletes, I see a huge variation of exercises done with medicine balls. To get you started I've gone into detail here about a couple of trunk-related exercises which I use regularly, but don't be afraid to innovate as your confidence grows. Just be careful: don't be stupid and injure yourself doing silly tricks for the sake of it.

First of all is the rugby (or lateral) pass: you can see from the pictures on this page that for this exercise you need a partner. Stand facing to the front (i.e. both facing the same way and not staring at each other) and using the rotation of the trunk throw the ball sideways to your partner. This should be done quite vigorously. You will need to be quite a distance apart to make the exercise effective. The idea is to keep your feet in position and really rotate from the obliques to get the momentum into the ball. Obviously you can increase the difficulty of the exercise by using a heavier ball and moving further apart. Try to be as accurate as possible with your throwing and keep the ball moving continuously – as you receive the ball use its momentum to pivot round to the opposite side of your body before reversing the movement fluidly and slinging it back.

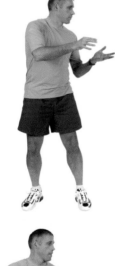

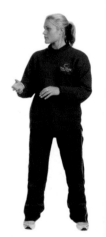

Obviously this is a great exercise for any sports where you will be using trunk rotations (tennis, golf and rugby, for example) and also as an alternative to the usual crunches you will get thoroughly sick of doing time and time again.

At a really advanced level you can do the same exercise sitting while balancing on an exercise ball – this is really tough and takes a huge amount of practice to perform with any kind of control or grace!

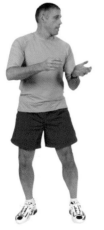

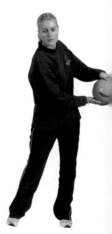

The photos on the right show a really strenuous trunk exercise that focuses on abdominals and hip flexors. You will need to be pretty strong in this area to start working on these exercises; use a 1 or 2kg ball at first before moving on to the heavy stuff.

You get ready in the normal trunk curl position (see page 178) but this time holding your arms out more or less straight behind your head with the ball in your hands. You then sit up, subtly bending the arms to assist the movement, and release the ball towards the top of the movement to your training partner to catch. If the ball just goes up and comes straight back down on your head it's a reminder that you've let it go too early! If, on the other hand, you throw it into your partner's shins all the time you are letting go too late and risking it coming back at you at high speed – so work on getting the release angle right.

As your partner catches the ball, they will throw it back into your outstretched hands (you're still sitting up at this point) and you then put your arms straight over your head and lower carefully to the start point and repeat. Make sure you fixate the lower back and hips well for this exercise to get the most out of it and never lock the feet under anything as this transfers most of the work to the legs, which is not the idea.

I like the versatility of training with a medicine ball. You can be creative by mimicking sporting movements and actions, using the ball as a form of resistance over and above what is usually encountered. Most of the training does require a basic level of conditioning. though, so think about putting a few weeks' training under your belt before getting stuck into this. We're only scratching the surface here of what can be done with the medicine ball – other techniques, including explosive throwing and catching for arms, shoulders and chest, can be tailored to fit your own sporting and individual needs. Just apply some lateral thinking, then get out there and start playing with your balls!

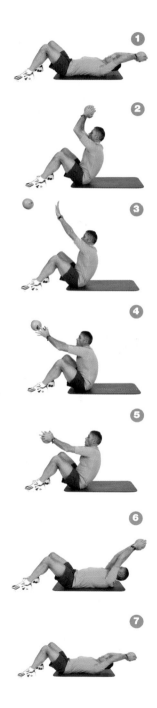

Good morning

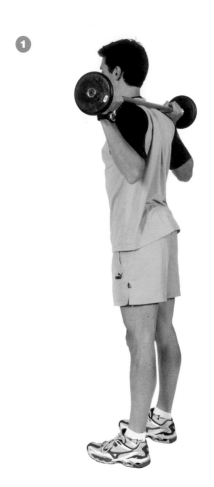

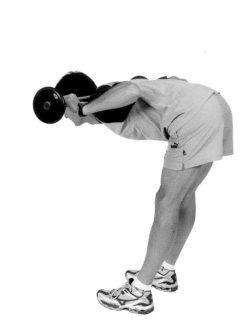

The good morning is an exercise that works the lower back, hamstrings and glutes.This is an exercise you need to be careful with because it's easy to get carried away with the weights. Always err on the side of caution with the amount of weight you can carry on the pivot point of your back. A good idea is to practise first with very low weights on the barbell or maybe even an unweighted broomstick.

Stand upright, looking forward and then lean forwards to approximately 50 or 60 degrees, but no more. Be aware of the limits of your flexibility; don't overextend and keep the movement forwards restrained. Your feet should be flat on the floor with all the pressure going through your heels. At the lower position, count 'one-two' and then come back up, but don't spring back up too quickly or aggressively. Control is the key word –

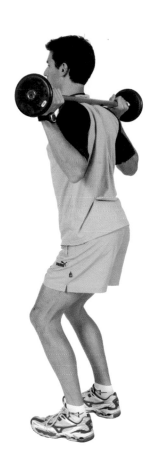

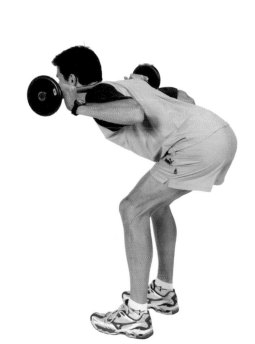

you will find that there is a lot of pleasure to be gained from the technique and control of this exercise.

It can be performed with straight or slightly bent legs, as shown in the pictures above. The bent leg variation is favoured for people with less flexibility in their hips and hamstrings.

I'm not entirely sure why it's called 'good morning' – it could be because it looks like the butler at Shrosbree Towers greeting us each morning.

Bernie's tip
Make sure you are well warmed up for this exercise. Some light, dynamic leg stretches are a good idea after an aerobic warm-up to get the range of movement in place before you load up the weights.

The legs

- **Step-ups and squat jumps • Lunges**
- **Calf raises • Machine and agility exercises**

VERY RARELY IN MY LIFE HAVE I GONE to a gym to work specifically on my legs. I'm lucky, because most of the sports that I enjoy – hill running, cycling and skiing, for example – are great for building up leg strength anyway. In fact, of all the parts of the body, our legs are probably the ones which even the least fit of us will find are in relatively decent condition, simply because we walk on them most of the time without thinking about it. Just work out how many miles you put in a week pacing around the office, pushing that trolley round the supermarket or walking the dog! To the sports scientists, that's

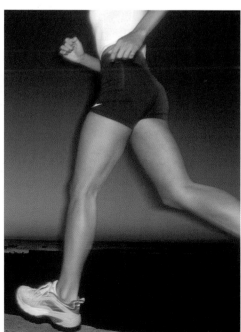

locomotion. To you and me it's simply walking, although walking upright is what separates us from most of the rest of the animal kingdom...

If I'm doing circuit training then I will be using my legs through the dynamic exercises that circuits involve. The exercises on the following pages are invaluable if you are trying to recondition your muscles, or doing some rehab after an injury – and it's amazing how many leg-related injuries occur. Just because we use our legs every day doesn't mean they are indestructible.

The danger is that you can assume that your legs are strong, start doing a bunch of heavy squats in the gym, and suddenly your knees pop. Writing and thinking about these exercises has made me realise that the muscle groups in the leg are absolutely critical to overall conditioning and performance.

Many sports obviously need leg strength just to be able to perform at any level – running or cycling, say – but if you are serving at tennis you need power from the legs, and if you are a shot putter a great deal of the explosive power comes from your lower limbs too. Follow the exercises in this section carefully and you should see the benefits, working up through initial conditioning to specific work on the quads, calves and hamstrings.

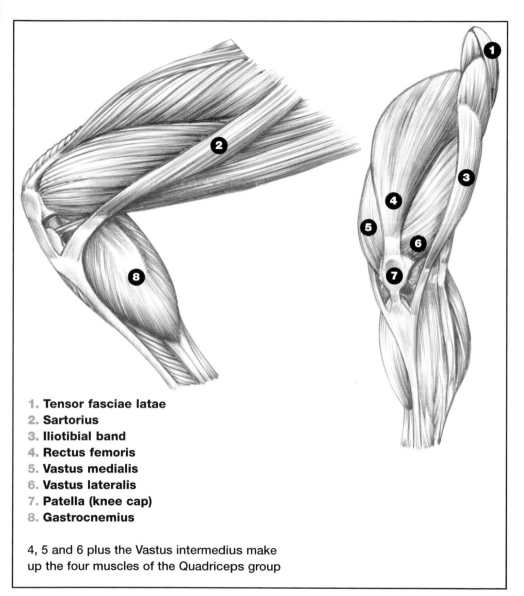

1. **Tensor fasciae latae**
2. **Sartorius**
3. **Iliotibial band**
4. **Rectus femoris**
5. **Vastus medialis**
6. **Vastus lateralis**
7. **Patella (knee cap)**
8. **Gastrocnemius**

4, 5 and 6 plus the Vastus intermedius make
up the four muscles of the Quadriceps group

Bernie's tip
We all tend to take our legs for granted but time spent conditioning this group of muscles will
really benefit your performance in just about every sport, particularly if you have not participat-
ed in a while and don't want to get silly injuries by blasting straight back into competition.

Step-ups
and squat jumps

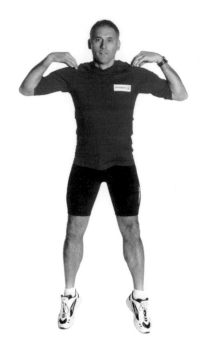

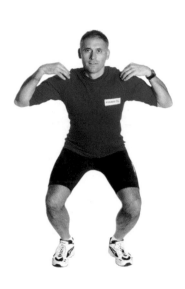

The step-up (right) allows you to work one leg at a time, so that you don't favour one side over the other, and is a good component for any circuit training programme. It also increases the range of movement in your hip area. You can perform it with dumbbells or a barbell for added resistance. And if you want to concentrate on one leg in particular – the push-off leg for a hurdler, triple jumper or high jumper – then you can do several reps on that one leg at a time. Otherwise, alternate the stepping legs.

The higher the bench the harder the exercise becomes. Complete the full range of movement by standing tall on the step for each rep – not just doing half steps, as you won't do yourself justice cheating like that.

The squat jump (above) is a demanding plyometric exercise – one of my favourites – that is another circuit training staple, really working your CV system. A plyometric exercise utilises something called the 'stretch shortening cycle' in a muscle. The theory is that by dynamically stretching a muscle immediately prior to a powerful contraction, greater explosive force can be generated.

Always remember to use a mat or a spring floor; never work on a hard floor or concrete because of the massive explosive power going through the knees.

Don't squat down too low – 90 degrees is plenty – and don't pause between jumps. Keep it going to get that plyometric effect working. Focus on a fixed point to stop yourself migrating across the gym into another person while you are doing a set.

Great for developing explosive power – you'll be whistling up some long-time dormant muscle fibres on these exercises.

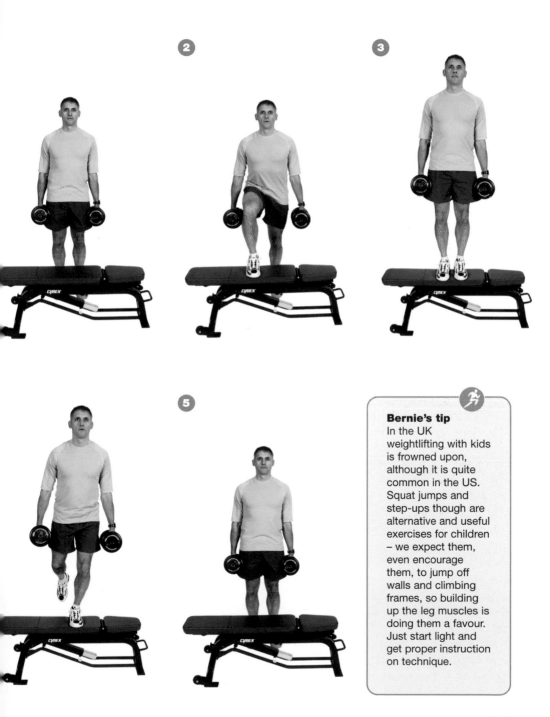

Bernie's tip
In the UK weightlifting with kids is frowned upon, although it is quite common in the US. Squat jumps and step-ups though are alternative and useful exercises for children – we expect them, even encourage them, to jump off walls and climbing frames, so building up the leg muscles is doing them a favour. Just start light and get proper instruction on technique.

Lunges

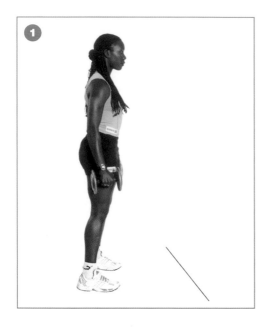

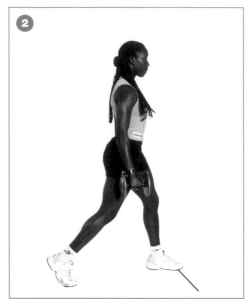

The lunge is a good, low-impact exercise that really works on your range of movement, particularly in the hip area. The movement, stepping forward and dropping down, works the hamstrings on the way down (as you bend your leg), and the quads on the way back up as you straighten the leg again. It's great for tennis and squash, and also for fencing, where the lunge is one of the most basic and effective moves.

In the start position you are standing feet shoulder width apart, making sure you are evenly balanced before beginning the lunge. Then step forward – a half step should be sufficient; you don't need to overextend. Keep your posture upright throughout.

As you land on your leading leg, drop your knee down to a comfortable position, ideally at a right angle to your leg. Never bend the leading leg more so that it is forming an acute angle; on the other hand, don't worry if the angle of your leg is more than 90 degrees, since we all have such different body shapes and mechanics. Try to keep the movement under control. Gravity will bring your body down, but don't just drop like a sack of potatoes.

Once you have reached the lowest position, push back up with an explosive return to the starting position. Use the toes on your leading foot to propel you back. The movement should feel like you are springing up.

Initially concentrate on a simple lunge forward, coming back to your original start point. You can put a marker on the floor to make sure you are lunging to the same point each time.

There are a couple of alternatives: you can do a walking lunge, where you come back up but rather than bringing your front

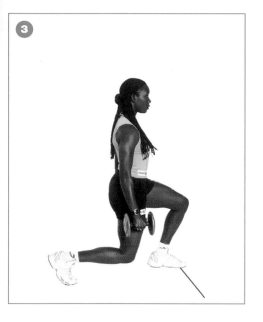

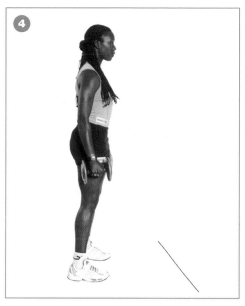

leg back to the rear leg, you move the rear leg forward to join the front leg, so that you move across the floor – particularly good for sprinters. You can also lift your knee higher when you step forward, which will help tennis players learn to take a good wide step. Finally, you can add weights, a dumbbell in each hand or a barbell across the back of your shoulders (after a certain level of conditioning there's a limit to how much weight you can carry in your hands). The barbell will also help

you keep your posture good and upright; the weight behind you prevents you leaning forwards, which is a bad habit to develop.

This is a great exercise for racquet sports, like tennis or squash, dipping down low for those difficult-to-reach balls. The lunge will give you the flexibility to be there sooner rather than later. Add variations by stepping off to the left or right, rather than straight ahead.

Sarah's tip
You may find this exercise quite difficult because of the amount of balance you need. So practise it without weights until you are really confident and feel well balanced through the range of movement. It does take a fair amount of coordination.

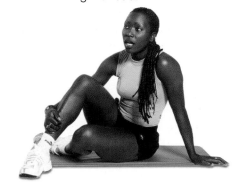

Calf raises

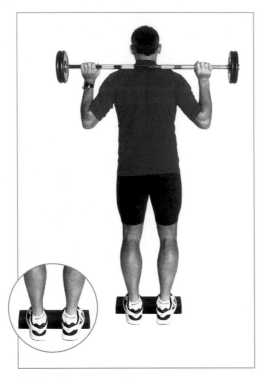

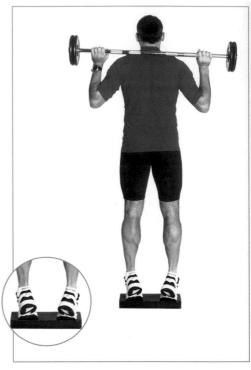

I try not to be negative about any form of exercise, but when it comes to calf raises I have to hold my hands up and say, 'What a boring exercise this is', possibly one of the dullest exercises ever invented. Some gyms have spent serious money buying in a specific calf raise machine – frankly you might as well play a pub piano. But, they do play their part in developing the calves for sports where toeing off is critical, such as high jump or racquet sports. And although running up a sand dune has exactly the same effect, not everybody has a handy sand dune at the bottom of the street. So, take no notice of me, and fit this exercise into your programme once in a while.

All you need is a block, about 4cm or so high. Make sure it has a good grip so that it won't move while you're standing on it. Use a barbell with some light weights and place it behind your neck on your trapezius. Rest the balls of your feet on the block (not your toes), and keep your heels on the ground. Then transfer your weight forwards and lift your heels off the ground, making sure you extend the ankle as much as possible. Keep the whole movement smooth and controlled. Don't tackle it too aggressively or your achilles tendons (which are the longest in your body) may just go snap. Preferably, though, hit the beach!

Personally, this exercise would bore me rigid – but I could run in the dunes all day, and achieve the same effect.

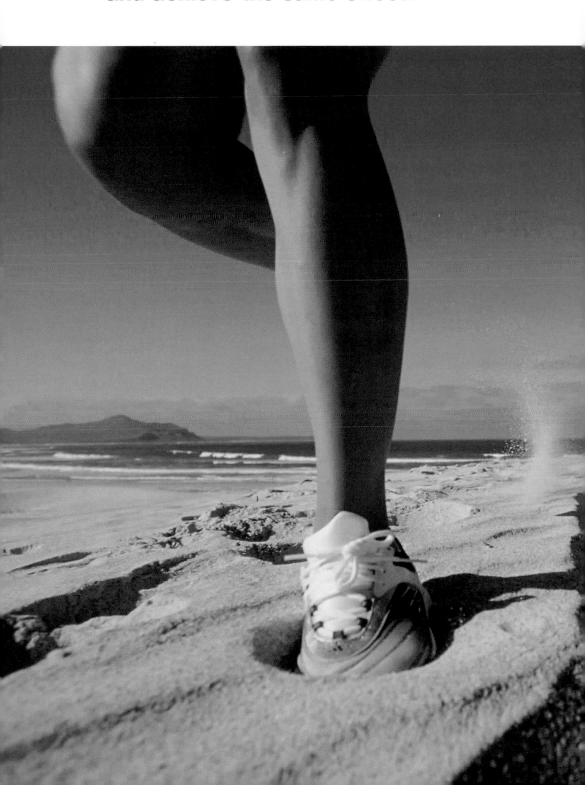

Machine exercises

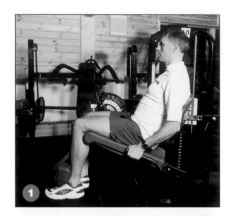

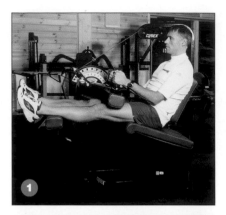

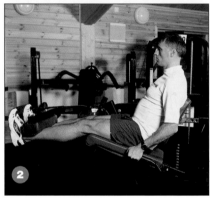

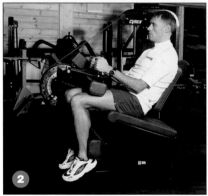

The leg extension (above) is working the quads, and the set-up is vital. To avoid overextending your leg (hyperextension), the cam should be set so that your leg stops just before full extension. Initially this was designed as a machine for rehab on a muscle following injury and although it is now in general use, that original purpose is its best use. Don't imagine that building up your quads will give you a stronger kick if you play football – that comes from the hip movement. Where the leg extension machine may be particularly useful is if you have a muscle imbalance, so you can work on one leg alone.

In the leg curl exercise (above), you are sitting on the muscle you are working. Check that, as on most modern machines, the seat height and the position of the leg pads is adjustable. If they are not, be careful that when you sit against the back pad there is no restriction preventing your legs pulling the lever down. This exercise will work your hamstring, which is a large muscle group, but extremely delicate (remember how often footballers limp off with a damaged hamstring). When a sprinter pulls up, it's usually because their quads are too powerful and the hamstring isn't up to the job of acting as the brake.

Although gym machines are good because they control the range of movement in an exercise, they can also be very dangerous if you don't get the set-up right.

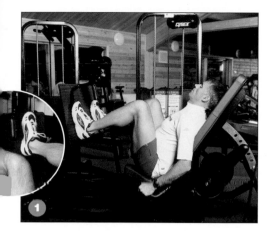

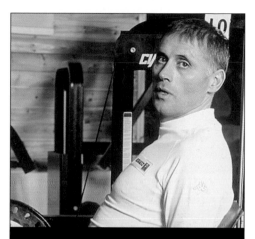

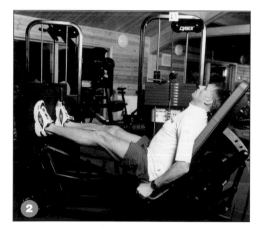

The leg press will mainly stress your quads but if you place your feet on top of the foot plate (see inset photo) you will place more emphasis on hamstring and glutes. This exercise is similar to the squat and is probably a better option if you have back problems or are starting a strength programme. Pay particular attention to the set-up of the machine. Do not allow the knees to be flexed to less than 90 degrees and do not totally lock the knees out on full extension.

It's so easy to walk into a gym that looks like the shopfloor in an engineering works, and imagine that everything is ready to go. Make sure you have a proper induction before leaping onto the equipment. Listening to inductions is very important; an injury will only occur if you don't follow the rules. I am very tough on this; if somebody in my team doesn't check the cam set-up when working with someone who is new to a machine, I give them a right earful. Do be careful in a new gym. You can't always assume that the instructors have been properly instructed themselves. If the induction feels rushed or doesn't tell you what you want to know, maybe you need to change gyms. Trust your instincts; you wouldn't do a parachute jump after ten seconds of explanation. If you have any doubts, review the club rather than risk your body's health.

Agility exercises 1
Hexagonal jumps and hurdle jumps

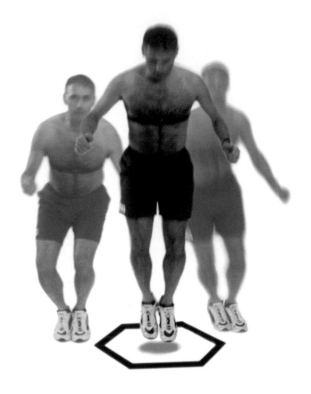

The hexagonal jump requires a high level of range of movement by everything from the hips downwards. It's demanding on your cardiovascular system, as well as working your hips, quads and calves, and another combination exercise that is good for any sport that requires quick changes of direction from lateral to forward or backward movement: a rugby side-step, soccer, all the racquet sports. Practising in the gym will bring you significant rewards on the playing field or squash court. I've used this with hefty 18-stone rugby players who previously had no idea what 'light on your feet' meant; after a few sessions they could be out there in a tutu…

You need to mark out a hexagon on the floor of your gym or home exercise area, with each side approximately 50cm long. You can do this with some masking tape or cut a shape out of card.

Then stand in the middle, facing forward, and toe off, springing out of the hexagon and back in, moving in each of the six directions in turn, but always facing forwards. Go clockwise round the hexagon, then change direction.

The key here is to be fast but precise with your movements. Try to land bang in the centre of the hexagon and only jump just outside the lines – it's no good being really powerful and fast but not really in control of your flailing limbs. Remember, 'Power is nothing without control.'

Keep as light on your feet as possible: think Rudolf Nureyev rather than Nelly the Elephant. You don't want to leave a crater in the ground.

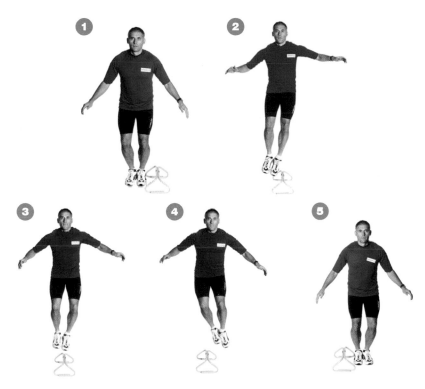

The hurdle jump (above) also needs a good continuous rhythm. The jump is over a small plastic hurdle or a low foam block, but the height of the obstacle is not the important thing (certainly it shouldn't be any higher than 10cm). Whatever you use make sure it is not a solid block because if you land on it when you are starting to get fatigued, you can easily damage an ankle. Keep your feet tight together, then take off across the hurdle and land with your feet together. Keep the movement swift and smooth. Remember to repeat the movement going back the other way and oscillate between each direction.

This is a great exercise for pre-skiing preparation in the autumn before heading for the slopes, as it builds up your quad and leg strength and replicates some of the movements of downhill skiing. Skiing is a very demanding sport from a physical point of view, and most once-a-year skiers don't really prepare enough. This exercise is one way to avoid coming back home with a plaster cast.

Bernie's tip
When you are doing the hexagonal jump try to minimise your contact with the ground. A study after the LA Olympics in 1984 revealed that the fastest sprinters were those who had the shortest amount of contact with the ground. That split second variation made all the difference.

Agility exercises 2
Lateral jumps

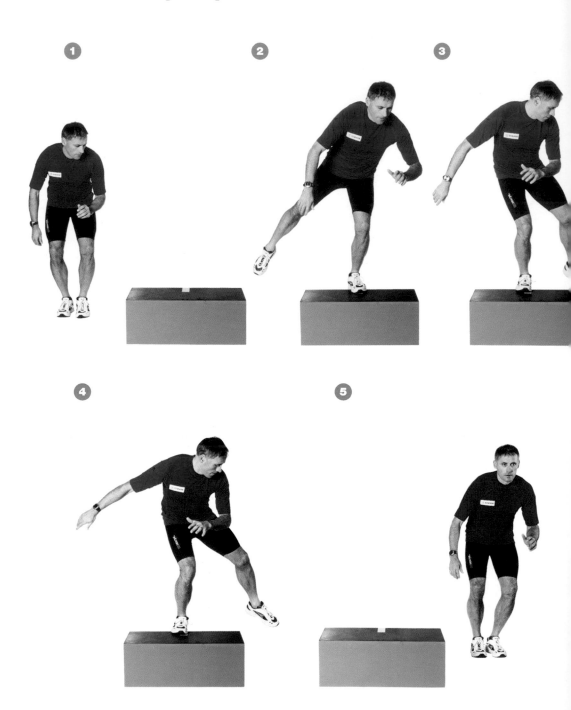

These exercises look simple. But they are both very demanding. Don't underestimate the balance required, or there will be tears.

I first came across the lateral jump in 1977 when I was involved in cross-country skiing. It was an exercise that the Scandinavians were using to improve both their skiing and skating skills. I liked it immediately and have used it ever since. It's fantastic for all-round leg conditioning for all field sports like hockey, rugby and soccer, and for the racquet sports. It's all about explosive power, and gives you great strength in your adductors.

You need to prepare the exercise first. Place the box you are using – and make sure it's strong enough to take the weight of you landing on it – and mark the centre point with some tape. That will be the target for your jump. Also place markers on either side of the box for your starting and landing positions, so the movement in each jump is consistent and controlled.

Stand with soft knees ready to explode off the ground, then toe off, springing off your outside foot to land on your other foot just beyond the centre mark on the box, then immediately transfer your weight onto the outside leg as it joins the leading leg. Push off again to continue the movement across the box before landing on the floor with a squatting movement. The whole movement should flow continuously with no breaks and pauses. Practise it first in slow motion, so that your body gets to know the movements, before trying it at normal speed; it is quite a complex movement.

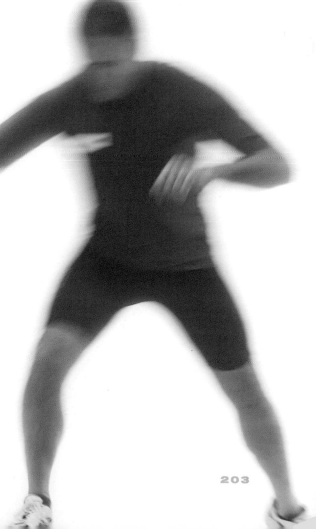

Bernie's tip
Make sure you've got a decent non-slip surface and good training shoes for these exercises. The consequences of slipping over might be more serious than just making a fool of yourself.

Warm-up, cool down and stretching

- Neck and shoulders • Forearms and abdominals
- Trunk and obliques • Hips • Lower back and
hamstrings • Quadriceps and calves

THERE ARE A NUMBER OF MYTHS I want to dispel about warming up, cooling down and stretching. These terms, particularly warm-up and stretching, are frequently used interchangeably, despite having very different meanings. Also, warming up and stretching are often spoken about as 'basic' elements of training – and I guess that they are once you have an understanding of them, although it's amazing how many people don't.

There was a time, years ago, when what most people thought of as a warm-up for sport involved getting your leg up on a brick wall and bending your chin down to touch your toes. This was all thanks to TV and the spectacle of highly trained gymnasts contorting their extremely elastic bodies. People thought that this was the right way to 'limber up'.

Thankfully, since then, a certain amount of common sense has prevailed, especially as nowadays most of us lack even a basic level of mobility. In the 1960s and 1970s people still used to walk or ride a bike to work. Now it's straight into the car for anything from a ten-minute to a two-hour commute. Our bodies are simply less used to being agile, and so are even more susceptible to damage caused by either any sudden or extreme movements or if we fail to prepare for exercise properly. Despite this, I still go into health clubs or watch league soccer on

Sundays, and find people trying out incredibly contorted stretching movements, without, I suspect, understanding exactly what it is they are trying to achieve. If you ask people to 'warm-up', a lot of them will still do a couple of side bends and then touch their toes, even though stretching is, in most cases, an activity to do after training or as a training session in its own right. It's a common misconception that static stretching, as practised by runners who stick a leg up on the wall before going for a run, somehow prepares the body for a jog even though there's no real reason to do it – it's just part of a routine or ritual, something they've always done! Sprinters, and particularly hurdlers, might do some stretching before their training sessions and races but this is very specific to their sport and highly dynamic, with high leg kicks and ballistic movements, not the stretch and hold for twenty seconds that most people might expect. Scientists and top coaches now reckon that static stretching actually reduces the power produced by a muscle immediately after the stretch. It causes a protective reflex to reduce pressure on the tendons by lowering the number of muscle fibres recruited (hope you took all that in!). In summary, avoid static stretching before you go out and train; save it for later!

Before you start warming up, you need to have some idea about the basic

Remember, there was only one Olga Korbut. Stretching and warming up doesn't mean having to tie yourself in knots.

principles, of what's actually going on in your body when you prepare for your sport. My motto is, 'If you don't understand it, don't do it.' If my car goes wrong I lift up the bonnet and if I can't immediately see the problem, I leave it to an expert mechanic. An awful lot of people 'lift up the bonnet' on their bodies and are convinced that they know what they are doing. Usually they haven't got a clue, but believe they should already know about warming up and stretching and so are afraid to ask about it because they think it is 'obvious'. I always say the opposite: 'Ask the dumb question – it's probably the most important you'll ever ask.'

The main reasons for warming up the body are to start creating a blood flow to your muscles; to raise the temperature of the muscles; to get your engine (heart and lungs) going; and to fire up the muscle fibres and nerve endings you'll be whistling up when you start really going for it. You are also getting your mind focused on the task in hand. Warm-ups are essential for anyone, but become more and more important as you get older – just like an old car which needs starting early on a cold morning. You can also think of your muscles as like a piece of Blu Tack. If it is old and has been lying around for a while it will break straight away if you try to stretch it. However, if you put it in your hand and warm it up for a while, then gradually stretch it a little, release it, and then stretch it a little further, you will be able to stretch it a long way without it snapping. This works in the same way as the elastic components of your muscle fibres as they age. That's why if you throw yourself straight into a

deep lunge to 'warm yourself up' without any preparation you will simply create a mass of microtears in your muscles. All you will be doing is helping yourself to get injured. You might just as well call the physio before you start – so he can be there quicker.

If I'm heading out of the front door for a run first thing in the morning, I avoid any static stretching, especially if I've got straight out of bed. All you need to do is swing your arms, moving them in a circle in front of you while keeping them bent. Do a few gentle high knee lifts, flex your ankles, shake out your legs and jump up and down on the spot. Basically you are mobilising just your joints and peripheries. Then it's into a walk, followed by a jog. If you rush out of your front door pressing your stopwatch without any preparation, the only thing you'll be timing is how quickly you can get injured.

If you are going out for a run take the climate into account. We've all seen those runners slogging around in the winter just wearing a vest and shorts. That is not hardy, just foolhardy. On the other hand, you don't have to overcompensate by bagging yourself up in layers of plastic, like a mobile garbage bag waiting to be picked up by the bin man. That's at the other end of the scale, the school of sweat – which merely dehydrates you. If the weather is cold, particularly make sure that you are wearing leggings, as your muscles are very susceptible to damage if they are cold.

The other thing that people often do is to walk straight onto a squash court for a lunchtime match and start smashing the

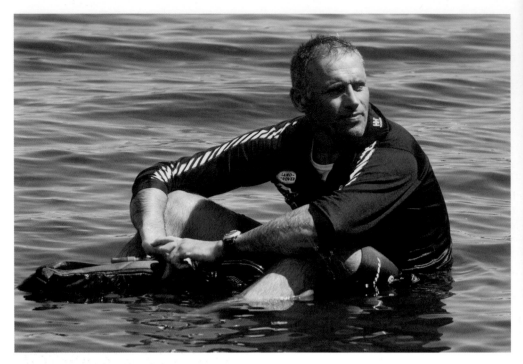

ball against the back wall as hard as they can, without any attempt at preparation. Even a few moments spent simply swinging your racquet or some light mobility and jogging will help move your blood to where it is needed and reduce the injury risk. I'm amazed at the effort that goes into optimising the ball's performance by warming it up whilst players neglect their own bodies!

After a session, the nature of 'the cool down' (not the warm down, which some people call it, and which is just a meaningless phrase) will depend on the intensity of the activity you have just completed. If you have been doing a heavy cardiovascular session on a rowing machine you need to cool down with an active recovery exercise; don't just collapse onto a mat. I like to have a nice, easy spin on a bike, or walk gently until my heart rate has come down; if I am outdoors a light jog is good. Once your

heart rate has dropped down to about 120bpm or below, take some fluids, and then do some mobility and a range of movement exercises for 10 to 20 minutes.

The area of cooling down is one of the most talked-about aspects of exercise, but is frequently one of the most neglected. Make sure you find the time to do it. Build into your programme a five-minute low-intensity spin on a bike or on the rowing machine before your shower. But that doesn't mean having a shower is optional. You should always shower after a workout, not just for reasons of hygiene, but because of the beneficial effect of warm water on your muscles. If you want to, you can also have a sauna to relax.

Whatever you choose to do, make sure you relax. The calming down process is as important as the actual cooling down. Don't just train for the session. Think to yourself while you're relaxing, 'What was that session all about, what did I gain

After a 10-hour day on the Mark Webber Tasmanian Challenge, a soak in cool water soothes aching limbs and invigorates sore muscles

from it?' Debrief yourself mentally while you are cooling down physically. When you have completed your exercise, this is the time to do plenty of work on your range of movement and flexibility. This is particularly important if you have played a ferocious game of squash or tennis or have finished a dynamic speed circuit. Instead of rushing off to the showers, set aside some time for range of movement work. It helps to ease out the muscle fibres and rearrange them from the stressful series of contractions you've been putting them through. In a sport like cross-country skiing, for example, where I was doing three sessions of training a day, it was vital for me to spend time doing some good range of movement, otherwise I would pay dearly later on. Cross-country skiing is all about technical skill and balance in the glide phase, which can go straight out of the window if you're still stiff and sore from the previous session.

If your time is genuinely tight, you can do this post-exercise stretching and range of movement work at home in front of the TV, in which case you need to treat it as an additional session. Just remember that you will need a small warm-up again to get your muscles ready for the stretch.

It is worth noting that top athletes, particularly sprinters, will devote whole training sessions to warming up, stretching to increase or maintain their range of movement, and then cooling down! Most of the rest of the world sees this as an unnecessary option at the end of a training session: I hope you will now realise why it is so important.

One question I often get asked is, 'How much warming up do I need?' This obviously depends on the kind of activity you're about to do but generally shorter, more intense activities require longer, more intense warm-ups than steadier sessions. If you are about to start a light cardio-vascular session the warm-up does not need to be very dynamic. But if you are about to do some powerlifting or a 100m sprint, your warm-up should build up to be accordingly explosive. If you are walking onto a football pitch, you may be required to perform some dynamic movements early on, and if you are not warmed up properly you will be putting yourself in danger of microtears and injuries. Take a considered view about the level of intensity you need. If it's even relatively high, you will probably want to make sure a professional coach is advising you. Top sprinters, whose events last as little as six seconds, will often warm-up for up to two hours or so before competing, much longer than marathon runners for instance. If they ran for two hours before racing they would just use up valuable energy stores! You're more likely to see them doing some light mobility and jogging, followed by a handful of pick-ups at race pace before heading to the starting line ready to go, all of which probably doesn't take more than half an hour.

Stretching from head to toe

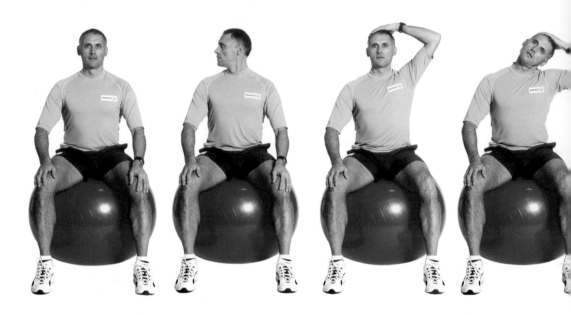

There are whole books devoted to stretching exercises. The ones I have picked out here are some basic stretches which will work out most parts of your body. Try them all out and find which ones come easily, and which ones are difficult for you. That way you will discover your strengths and weaknesses in terms of range of movement.

These exercises appear in this book as part of the cooling down process, which means that you gain most benefit from performing these stretching exercises when your muscles are warm and have been worked well beforehand. They are not designed to be used from cold, so don't go into the gym and launch straight into a series of vigorous quad stretches because you see everyone else starting their session like that.

Here I am showing the basic process of static stretching that is the most commonly used form of flexibility training. There are other more advanced techniques such as PNF (see the side bar on page 217) or ballistic stretching that top athletes use, but these require professional instruction as there is a higher risk of injury.

For these static stretches, look to hold a comfortable stretch for 10 to 20 seconds for each muscle group and repeat that two to three times in any one session.

I like to do a range of stretching exercises which work down from the head and then out to the extremities. Most of these stretches can be done from standing or seated positions.

Neck and shoulders

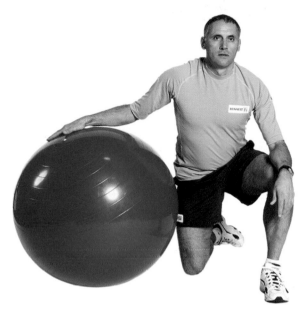

In sports like squash or football you will be making a lot of head movements, but over-dynamic head rotation or cycling the neck in training can be dangerous. In the exercise shown to the left, sit on the ball, keep your shoulders square and simply turn your head left, look back to the front, and then to the right. To increase the stretch, place your hand on your head and push down to one side.

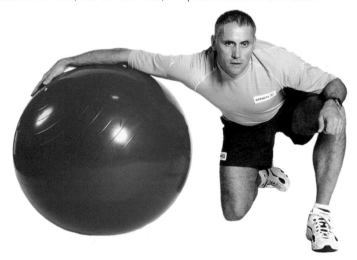

For the shoulder area, sit down next to the ball, with the outside leg bent at the knee and in front of you as shown in the top photo.

Stretch out your shoulder by rolling the ball away to the side holding the stretch and then rolling the ball back to the start position.

Upper back, shoulder and upper arms

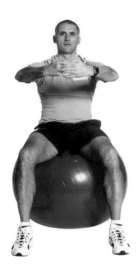 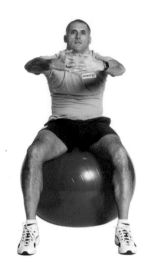

This is called 'hugging the mother-in-law'! I'm not sure how politically correct that name is, but it's a great description of how this exercise, which stretches the upper back region, is performed. Sit on the ball and put your arms out straight, interlocking the fingers with your palms facing your chest. Keep your elbows parallel with the floor, and then push your arms away from you keeping your body upright. You should feel the stretch across your upper back.

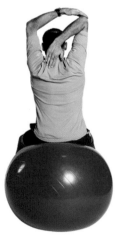 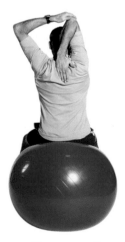

Now let's move onto a stretch for the upper arms. Reach behind your head with one arm as shown and gently press down on its elbow with your other hand to increase the stretch. Keep an upright posture, whether sitting or standing.

Forearms and abdominals

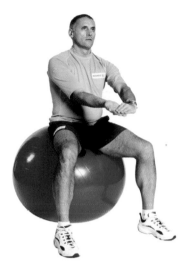 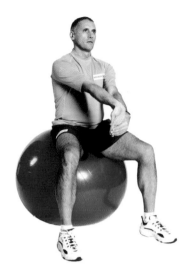

To finish stretching the arms, either sitting or standing, extend your arms out in front of you, parallel to the floor with your palms facing up. While keeping the arm level, push the fingers of one hand down towards the floor with the other hand, as above. This will stretch the forearm flexor muscles and feels fantastic if you have been using a lot of grip strength to lift heavy weights, for example.

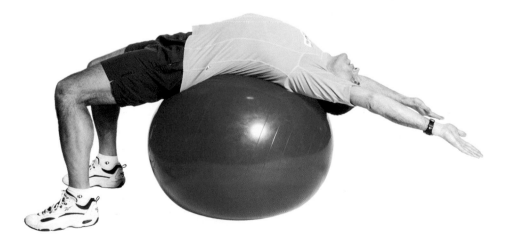

To stretch the abs after a hard workout or a circuit with lots of trunk work, stretch out with your back over the ball extending your straight arms towards the floor behind you. Reach back as far as you can to feel a stretch in your abdominal region.

Trunk and obliques

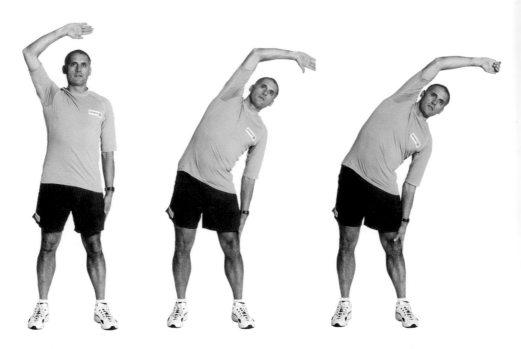

In this exercise the trunk and obliques will get a really good stretch. Begin by sliding your hand down to one side of your body while keeping the hand in light contact with your thigh.

You will immediately feel the stretch in both the hip and obliques on the opposite side. Hold the stretch at the end of your comfortable range of movement.

As your flexibility improves, you can increase the stretch, if (as in the photos above) you raise your other hand up above your head to do this. Make sure the quality of your technique is good by using a mirror to observe your shape.

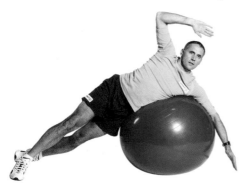
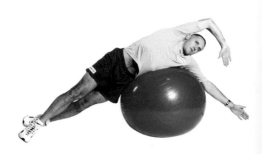

As shown above, you can also use an exercise ball to support your body weight throughout this exercise if you prefer.

Hips

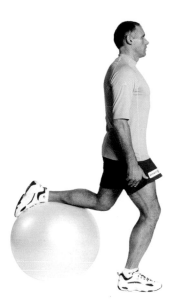

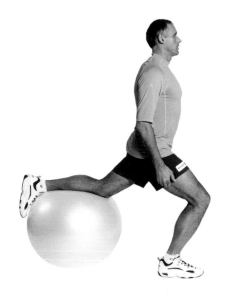

The hips are an area of the body where a lot of people find they experience tightness. These exercises will help you to stretch your hip flexors.

Using the exercise ball makes this easier if you find that your hips are stiff. The ball moulds itself into the shape of your lower leg, and helps you to control your range of movement by rolling the ball as far as is comfortable, and then gradually increasing the distance you roll it away.

In the other variation (below), keep your back knee on the floor – with a soft pad underneath it. Balance by keeping the front leg, which should bent at about 90 degrees at the knee, out to one side by 4–6 inches. Keep your upper torso straight. Place your hand into the small of your back, and push that hand (which should be flat) into the small of the back. Then walk the front foot forwards. For an advanced variation, bring the foot of your back leg up and push again.

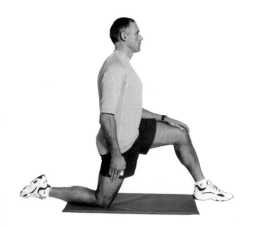

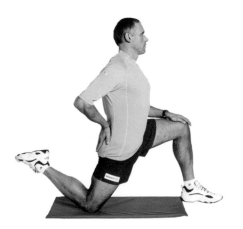

Lower back and hamstrings

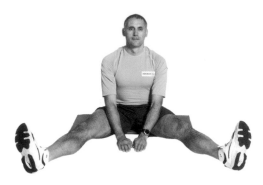

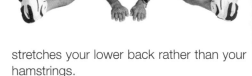

If you have been doing any kind of intense running or have been playing sports that involve dramatic changes of direction, like hockey or football, you need to stretch your hamstrings.

Sit on the floor with your legs apart, keeping your hands on the floor in front of you. If you are tight in your hamstrings and lower back, you will find that your legs will be slightly bent and your fingertips will only just touch the floor. If so, just draw your toes back and you will feel your hamstring stretch.

Try to get both your legs and hands flat on the floor; as you practise this exercise the range of movement in your hamstrings will increase. You want to avoid bending your legs, other than a very slight bend, as you lean forwards, because that just stretches your lower back rather than your hamstrings.

Once you find the movement is becoming easier, you can move your hands further forwards, eventually aiming to get your elbows onto the floor. In advanced, supervised training, you may see a trainer or helper leaning on the back of the person exercising, but this is done in a very controlled way. Don't get carried away and ask your chum to sit on your back.

In the other exercise (below), you draw one leg into the other thigh and then slide both hands down the straight leg over the knee. This is an advanced, combination stretch of both the lower back and hamstring, and is particularly good for sports like sprint hurdling.

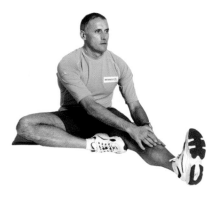

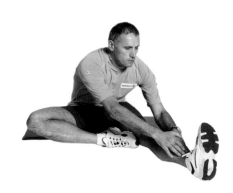

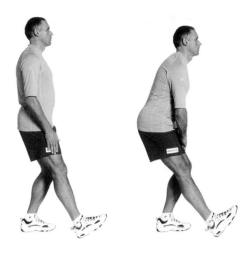

Place one foot out in front of the other, keeping that leg more or less straight, and your back foot flat on the ground. Retaining a soft bend in your back knee, place both your hands onto the thigh of the back leg and then make as if to sit down on a stool just behind you. Then lift the toe of your front foot. You will feel your hamstring stretch. Take it to the point where you feel the muscle is under tension but you are not in any pain.

Once you find that this exercise is not, well, stretching you, then you can increase the level of intensity by leaning slightly forwards as you make the movement. If your muscles, following a period of regular stretching, become more flexible, you can graduate to placing your front foot up on a higher surface, maybe on an exercise ball as shown below, but be very cautious about attempting this.

If you are cooling down in a group – with the rest of your football team, for example – you can fall into the trap of trying to copy the range of movement of the other guys who are training with you.

Each of us has an individual and different level of range of movement. So don't worry about anyone else's range of movement. Just concentrate on your own.

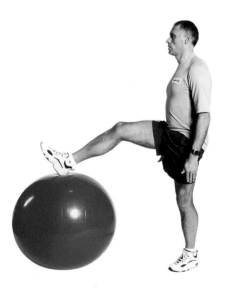

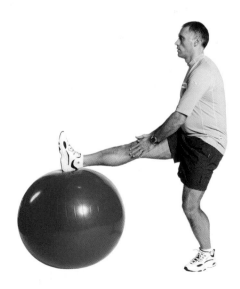

Quadriceps and calves

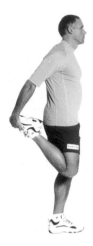 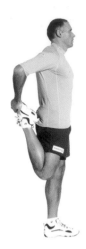

Fold one of your legs behind you at the knee by taking hold of the foot and pressing the heel into your backside. Either support yourself with the other hand against a wall, or keep your front knee soft if you have no support.

It is tempting to pick up your foot and then lean forward. Avoid this as you will not be stretching the muscle correctly. Keep an upright posture, pushing your hips forward to increase the stretch. If you are very stiff, and find this stretch difficult, an alternative version is to lie face-down on the floor, placing a towel around the leg behind you and using the towel to pull it towards your backside. Or use an exercise ball (as shown below), which can help if you have poor balance or if you have limited range of movement. The ball takes the place of your hand so that you can still stretch out your quads.

Finally, here is an exercise to stretch your calf muscles. There are two muscles that make up the calf – the gastrocnemius and the soleus – which need to be stretched independently. The basic start position for both stretches is the same. Stand facing a wall while placing both hands out in front of

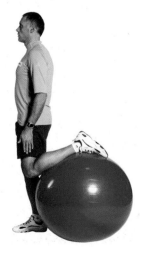 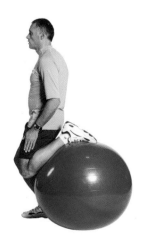

Always keep your breathing nice and relaxed. Don't become a member of the ugly club, who hold their breath when stretching and slowly go purple.

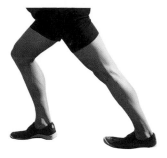

you at head height. To stretch the gastrocnemius, lean into the wall pushing one leg out behind you, keeping that heel firmly on the floor with the leg straight. Lean more into the wall and feel the upper calf stretch. Your front leg bends at the knee and provides balance, but most of your body weight should be supported by the back leg and your arms.

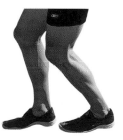

To stretch the soleus assume the original start position with your hands against the wall, but bring the back leg into a more forward position than for stretching the gastrocnemius; lean into the wall and bend the knee of the back leg. You will then feel the stretch lower down in the calf muscle, around the area of the achilles tendon.

If you work your way through all the exercises in this section you will have stretched your whole body, from your head through your trunk and torso to the ends of your arms and legs.

At the start of this section I mentioned PNF as an example of an advanced stretching technique. PNF stands for Proprioceptive Neuromuscular Facilitation! Now that's one to impress your mates with down the gym. It is an advanced stretching technique only carried out by an experienced physio or sports therapist. When you stretch and hold a muscle for a period of about 8–10 seconds or more it gradually relaxes as the elements in the tendon that recognise and prevent further stretching (to stop the muscle from tearing) are overridden. This is what you do in normal static stretching – quite effective for maintaining flexibility. However, PNF techniques take you to this point and then get you to contract the muscle you are stretching but without letting it shorten significantly (i.e. the physio holds the joint in place so that you perform a static contraction). This again stretches the same protective elements in the muscle that slowly relax and allow the physio to push the muscle a little further and produce a more effective stretch. This is generally acknowledged to be one of the best ways to improve flexibility quickly, but it goes without saying that this is not something to get your mate to try to help you with as you might end up being wheeled into Casualty shortly after hearing a nasty ripping sound. Leave it to the experts!

Enjoying the environment

I DON'T THINK IT'S AN EXAGGERATION to say that I owe my career success as a sportsman to the way I've learnt to embrace and overcome the physical and mental challenges that the great outdoors has thrown at me, as I've trained and competed over the years. The outdoor environment presents an always changing, always unpredictable set of tests, from extreme weather conditions, huge variations in temperature and humidity to massive varieties of terrain. And the rewards for thinking about how to go about tackling these elements as they

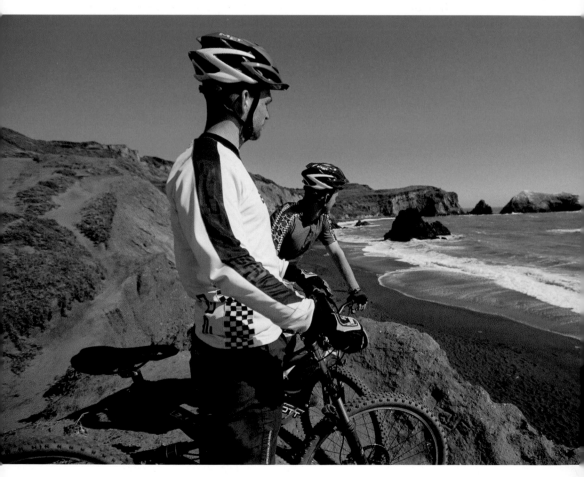

present themselves, coupled with the real conditioning and fitness benefits they can deliver as you hit the trail or climb onto the mountain bike, make them truly worth the effort of seeking out.

To give you some idea what I'm talking about you must know that feeling when, maybe while on a vacation, you step outside and start a leisurely walk or hike along a forest trail. The air is fresh and the conditions are perfect; and that feeling wells up inside that you are just plain glad to be alive, right? Well, what I have always tried to do, as a professional sportsman, is to take that feeling to a whole new level by actively challenging the environment.

If we are honest with ourselves, most of us spend a great deal of energy competing with other people – at work, home or even on the squash court – which is often a complicated and stressful business. The environment, though, is just there and it does what it does; inanimate maybe, although it doesn't always feel like it. I know a beach where the sea usually comes crashing in with a high surf. It is a mighty challenge to swim out against, and almost every time I try I end up washed up onto the beach, frustrated and laughing, saying, 'the bastard's beaten me again, I can't get out there'. But I love the challenge of attempting to fight and win over this particular environment. It's a great game to try to read and feel the water, working out how I can swim hard and efficiently, getting out beyond that big surf. And once I am out there in the gently rising and falling sea beyond the surf, I feel both physically and mentally satisfied.

Now don't get me wrong, I fully accept that working out and exercising in a gym has many advantages, but maybe you could achieve the same results outdoors, and along the way gain all the benefits of training in the natural environment.

If you've spent hours running on a treadmill indoors in an airless studio, give yourself a break and put all that training to good use on a trail run. Not only will you have a chance to run through some great scenery, but you'll find that suddenly you're experiencing a very different kind of running: dancing along undulating paths, dodging rocks and ruts. It all adds up to a completely new challenge, and one that will help you get out of a different kind of rut: the uninspiring one of turning up in the same locker room and exercising on the same machines in the same enclosed space week after week.

Or, if you've been concentrating on accumulating thousands of metres on the rowing machine, get out on the water and try it for real. Leave the exercise bike behind – don't worry, it will still be there when you get back – and use one that actually moves forwards and can take you to new places.

I know I tend to use the word 'euphoria' a lot – but that's because I really believe that so many people who grind themselves down with guilt about not making their 'regular' session have never experienced the natural high of achieving an enhanced performance out of doors. No wonder that the prospect of another hour on the treadmill isn't exactly galvanising them to change their lives. If that sounds all too familiar, then this section is for you.

I am assuming, by the way, that having read this far, you are willing to change your life? If so here is another story from my early years: being British, swimming mostly means ploughing up and down indoor swimming pools, but I've been part of a team that's swum the Channel and love the changing sea state. You go down in the early mornings and it can be like a millpond; a few hours later it may well turn into a raging swell with very dangerous currents. The sea, in all its states, was an environment in which I spent a great deal of my time as a member of the Special Boat Services. Usually it was dark as we emerged from a submarine into 15ft swells and 8-knot currents somewhere in the North Sea so that we could climb and secure an oil rig. I can tell you, when I first took part in this type of mission I was deeply frightened. Believe me, a sea of that magnitude at night is no place for any sane human being – a truly horrible environment. But, through good conditioning, training and practice, and learning the skills of the job, I found I could deal with it. Then it became a challenge – to do it really well and, when we did, that in turn gave me a huge amount of satisfaction and at times not a little euphoria. So now I can take real pleasure in open water swimming and have also learnt a valuable lesson that there is tremendous excitement to be had in conquering challenging environments. And, while it's something of a cliché it is also a truism that 'knowledge dispels fear'.

Now I am not for one moment suggesting that you set about tackling potentially dangerous environments without adequate training and supervision, and I certainly do not recommend you take up the new extreme sport of oil rig climbing, but why not, for example, add a few days of cross-country skiing to your winter holiday plans? Technically demanding and an excellent endurance-building sport, it will also take you into some of the most beautiful snow-clad countryside imaginable.

The other thing which I believe is really important is to mentally leave everything behind when you change into your training gear. I've seen business people with their mobiles switched on and to hand when they're running or working out. Turn the bloody thing off, leave it in your locker. Run and forget everything, or better still, run and sort out your life. Convert any stress you may be feeling into positive thinking. It's amazing how, almost without realising it, a lot of the 'problems' you imagine you are facing manage to sort themselves out while you're out in the fresh air doing some training.

Of course, being out in the environment does not necessarily mean having to be out in wooded valleys or on Lakeland hillsides. I did a BBC interview recently and stayed overnight in a hotel in central London near to Broadcasting House. I got up nice and early, asked the guys at the front desk where the nearest green space was, and they pointed me towards Regent's Park. There I was at six in the morning, in a fabulous environment, surrounded by beautiful architecture, running and clearing my head. It gave me personally a completely new concept of the city, seeing it at this time in the morning, as yet untarnished by all the

There is simply nothing better than challenging yourself both physically and mentally in a wonderful environment.

traffic noise and fumes. I got back, showered, felt great and was ready for the demands of the day ahead – and that was all down to the quality of the environment.

If you're on holiday, there's even less excuse for not getting outside. You'll probably find that not only are there great natural spaces nearby – maybe some dunes, a seafront promenade, hills and mountains, parks – but also the facilities which will allow you to take advantage of them, whether that's a mountain bike hire shop or a running trail along the coast.

When you're on holiday, there's certainly no way you can use the 'I'm sorry, work's just too busy at the moment' excuse...

As I keep saying, you are the only one who can get yourself fitter and improve your performance. The only person you're making excuses to is yourself; you know those excuses are usually nonsense. It's funny how busy you find yourself when you need to get out in the morning for a cycle ride, but then you can always make the time for a lunch or a party...

What I am hoping is that by your

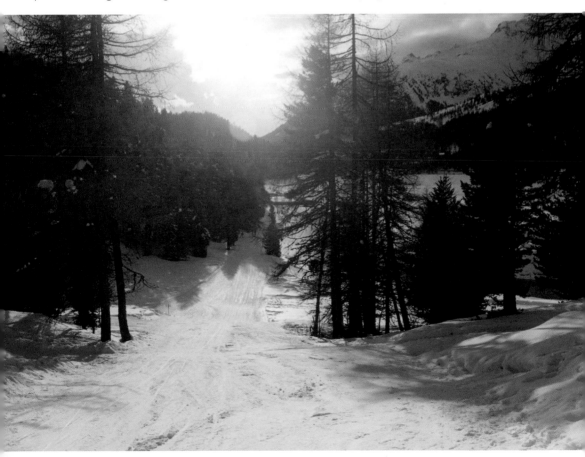

Virgin ski trails in St Moritz: they beat the gym any time

reading this, I will have succeeded in changing your attitude towards training and that you will be tempted to exchange the gym or fitness club for the outdoors – for at least some of the time. Get out there and learn new skills, learn to understand the environment you are in, and before long you will have a much-improved ability to work and train in it. And you will find a new level of enjoyment in the pursuit of your conditioning and sporting goals.

As you will have gathered, I love fell running and once, during filming of *Survival of the Fittest* in Snowdonia, we had really, and I mean really, bad weather – thunder and lightning, lashing rain, howling wind, the whole lot. It was so bad the television people couldn't fly their helicopters; they had to operate with a very limited camera crew and, in fact, there were people being taken off Mount Snowdon by the local rescue services. Our event that day was to run to the top of the mountain. Well I ran all the way to the top with a big Cheshire cat grin on my face. Why? Because I knew that the wind, the rain, the chill factor and the all-round physical discomfort was playing on other guys' minds, whereas here I was running in a euphoric state of mind – it's crazy, but that's what I like. And, in truth, it has given me a tremendous competitive advantage down the years.

What I often see is that people are simply ignorant about, or don't understand, the environment in which they are training or competing. We can be down at the base of a mountain talking about what a lovely mild day it is and how we are going to hike up to the top. But those who have never visited this sort of environment don't realise that when you get up near the summit at 3500m, there can be a wind chill of –5°C and probably sleet to snow or icy rain. Me, I love that because I am prepared mentally for the conditions. I know how I can deal with it. It's my day at the office and all I have to do is go to the filing cabinet, pull out the relevant file marked 'wet, windy and cold' and say, 'ah ha, we're working on this today'. I know, by opening that file that when the wind changes and the horizontal rain feels like someone's spraying you with a chilled garden hose, just what effect it all has on the body and how I can best deal with it.

Of course you can never win against the elements but you can compete against them to improve your own performance. I used to do a lot of white water paddling down extreme rivers, which, quite frankly, if you came out of your canoe would quite likely kill you. So what makes anyone want to do that? Well I won't deny that I really like to test myself. I can remember on one occasion when the water was a raging torrent; it just roared as I sat in my boat. The water towered above me and was so cold I had to wear ski clothes and half a dozen tops in an attempt to keep warm. There is a thing called breaking out which is when you leave an eddy and you get into this white foaming water, which is where I promptly capsized. Suddenly it all became a harsh, uncompromising and true test of skill; and a very scary moment. I had no doubt the river was trying to finish me off and that the best place to be was on top of it rather than underneath it. For

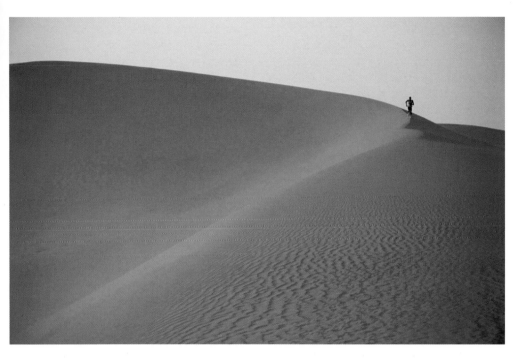

several minutes it was touch and go, but I was sufficiently experienced to win out and successfully negotiate the challenge.

Great experiences; they challenge your body, mind and soul. Perhaps that is what it is all about for me. Whether it's rock climbing, trail or mountain running, swimming in the open sea or paddling extreme rivers, I relish the raft of challenges each of these environments present. I enjoy the mental tests that the environment will always pose – so often there's a problem in front of you that is impeding your activity: a difficult overhang during a climb, a sharp turn you have to negotiate on 3cm skis, a sudden storm at altitude on a hike. Whatever it is, the aim for me is simple: to run the trail, climb the mountain and paddle the river.

The environment is so changeable that it offers you a new experience on a daily basis. I try never to be frightened by changing my routine – a lot of people seem to think that if they step one millimetre out of their training programme all hell will break loose. It's not like that. Use the programme as a way of structuring your exercise, but if the opportunity comes up for doing something complementary, then take it. Variety is the spice, and all that.

To be successful at getting fit, maintaining and improving that fitness, you have to go back to what may seem like mundane repetitions; that's the day job. But that's even more reason to enjoy the outdoors and the buzz you'll discover out there when you can.

Desert running in Libya: extreme, but what a challenge

Take it outside: but don't just go for a run – go for an experience.

At a training camp on Lanzarote, I went out for a run along a barren coastal ridge beside the sea. The weather was hot and humid, the terrain was rough, but the feeling of being outside watching these massive waves breaking on the rocks made me feel very, very good. If I'd been in a gym I would have felt OK, but I would not have felt the euphoria. Simply put, I felt like a kid again.

And when I was competing in triathlon on a regular basis, there were some winter mornings near my home in Dorset when I'd look at myself stuffed into eight layers of clothing to protect myself from the cold and wearing tights to keep my legs warm, and I'd think about my friends who were on training camps in California. It didn't matter to me – once I was up in the hills: with the frost on the grass and some sun cutting through the crisp air, I felt brilliant.

So what it all comes down to is this: where are you now? Yes you lot who are starting off on this great life-changing adventure, maybe down your local gym. And, as importantly, where can you take it? You could take it all the way to the level of a Pete Goss or even a Bernie Shrosbree, but what you've got to do is make sure you start this challenge, set your goals, make the commitment – then take it to the elements. Remember that using the environment will almost always make you feel better. Try it, and you'll suddenly find a whole new lease of fitness life. 'Don't just go for a run. Go for an experience.'

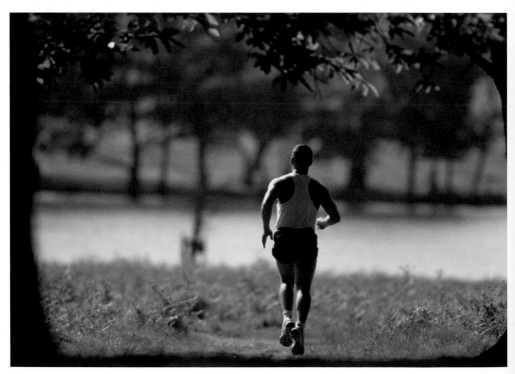

Challenging the environment and yourself *Pete Goss*

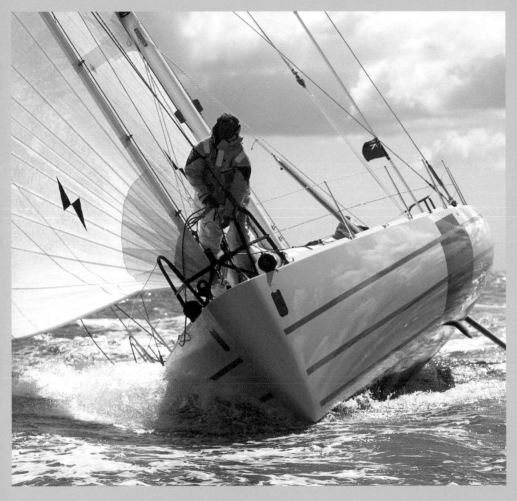

I first met Bernie in the Royal Marines when he joined our troop in Scotland. Straightaway he struck me as something of a kindred spirit and we hit it off immediately. Over the next few years I did a lot of physical training with Bernie; in fact he quickly got the troop under his wing, bringing a degree of sophistication and passion to our training we'd not experienced before, introducing us to skiing, running on the beach, canoeing, all sorts of new areas. By then Bernie had been in the Marine's biathlon team and was doing a lot of competitive running and it was about this time he was on the point of getting married, so we were always going through the running magazines looking for the races where you could win a washing machine or a television and so on. I remember there was a 20-mile race in Newcastle and for some reason the organisers offered the first person to cross the 10 mile mark a fridge, so Bernie trained for 10 miles, hit the wall, got his fridge then jogged the rest of the way to the finish line. He opened up a whole new world of training for a purpose!

The corps also introduced me to ocean sailing, an activity which really grabbed hold of me. I can remember sailing dinghies as a youngster and, in fact, made my first Channel crossing from Plymouth to Treguier, with my dad, when I was about 12. I can clearly recall the sense of achievement when we made landfall after what proved to be a hard trip, an adventure that, in its way, was as rewarding as finishing the Vendée Globe would prove to be twenty or so years later. The trouble is if you like searching for new horizons, once you've crossed the Channel then you want to cross the Atlantic, once you've crossed the Atlantic you want to go around the world and then you want to go round single-handed. If you have that sort of passion and you're lucky (and get a lot of support) then eventually you will end up taking on some of the adventures that I've been lucky enough to have a crack at. We have a saying in sailing that knowledge dispels fear and so over a period of time you will build up the knowledge at which point the sea stops being an alien environment. These days I'm as happy at sea as I am on the land and would say that I am an adventurer, and that sailing is the medium through which I have been getting my adventure.

I really enjoy the big, long ocean races which have very loose rules and which give me the opportunity to develop and employ innovative technological solutions – something I'm particularly interested in. These ocean-crossing races also demand that you work with the environment – don't fight the environment, work with it – treat it as a friend as much as anything.

Tackling the huge challenges that such a potentially hostile environment as the Southern Ocean can throw at you is not the same thing as being an out-and-out risk-taker, which is often the perception of what we do. If, by way of an analogy, you said to a mountain biker go from the top to the bottom of a mountain as quickly as possible, then a risk-taker would grab the first bike they could find and throw themselves down to an unpredictable, and possibly injurious, outcome at the bottom, whereas what we would do, and I do underline the word we, is: carry out a lot of research; get hold of the best bike we can find; quietly go a quarter of the way down the mountain, half way, three quarters, perhaps finding along the way that we need to develop better brakes or some other element of the technology. Only when we have gone through all of these incremental processes would we choose to leave the top of the mountain for the actual challenge – confident that we would far outstrip the suicidal time of the impulsive risk-taker and knowing we had created a new, innovative technology at the end of the challenge. We would also operate with a quiet sense of inner confidence in the project and, although it's often unseen, we would have woven a safety net, which should preclude the ultimate sacrifice. Only then would we head out into the journey. So when I go on these races, I am not worried about dying – the risk is there, but it's quite a small risk; we don't take risk, but we do embrace risk.

As a single-handed sailor I am always asked about loneliness. During the four and half months of the Vendée Globe, considered by many to be the world's toughest yacht race – a non-stop, single-handed circumnavigation of the globe – I didn't feel lonely, but I missed people, which is a very different emotion. As I set sail I didn't quite know what to expect, but I discovered that I was really happy out there. I can't see the sea as the enemy and I never feel as if I am fighting it – in any case you could never beat it. What you are really trying to do is work with it and although it doesn't have any emotion, it is not this kind of faceless thing.

The race itself felt like four and half years of life condensed into four and a half months. The highs are very heady and the lows can be quite crushing, so it has a real intensity to it. It all comes down to you and the elements, which have all sorts of faces; the sensation of being on top of a 30-foot wave, watching the bow drop off and just disappearing down a tunnel of spray is absolutely fantastic. People often moan about the cold and the wet, but the sailing far outweighs it. The Southern Ocean is awe-inspiring, invigorating –

the raw energy is simply breathtaking. To go somewhere where there aren't even aircraft vapour trails in the sky is fantastic and it can bring both the best and the worst out in you. I've come to the conclusion that it does you good to go out into the wilderness and get things into perspective. Once, I remember sailing the Atlantic at two o'clock in the morning in the trade winds, surfing along at 15 knots. There was a full moon and I'm sat on deck, with my personal stereo on listening to some jazz music, reading a novel – the moonlight was bright enough – and having two hundred dolphins start leaping around the boat with the moon reflecting across the bay. Everyone thinks that the ocean is this emotionless, grey frightening thing, but it's teaming with life and, frankly, mostly we don't know just what sort of animal life is out there. I've had killer whales jumping around the boat, flying fish on it, you see stars like you've never seen before, it's clean, it takes you back to your most basic self.

But when a big ocean does get up a bite, then you definitely find out what you have inside of you, and it can strip you to your very soul...

Christmas Day 1996, four months into the Vendée Globe, and the day had begun with a bright blue sky and a refreshing 20-knot wind from the north. I was 1,400 miles south of Perth, Western Australia and the only blot on the horizon was the rapidly falling barometric pressure. It was with a growing sense of foreboding that I checked everything on the boat Aqua Quorum, waiting for what promised to be a severe blow.

A few hours later I found myself in the worst seas I've ever encountered. Then as the boat was being repeatedly knocked down by huge waves, the SatCom system started bleeping. I managed to struggle across to the chart table – by now the boat resembled a yellow submarine – to discover that a Mayday had gone out from race control. A fellow competitor, Frenchman Raphael Dinelli, was in serious trouble. One look at the chart told me that Raphael was 160 miles away dead upwind, and to reach him I'd have to turn around and sail into the teeth of the atrocious storm. I had no choice of course; the decision to turn around was already made for me – many years ago by the tradition of the sea. When someone is in trouble you go to his or her aid.

Although I'd been involved in a number of rescues over the years, what confronted me now was both sobering and frightening. I sat myself down and began to think about what was to come and the possible consequences. I reflected on the important things in my life; my family, my boat and, of course, the risk to my own life. It seems to me that if you keep chipping away at life you will eventually come to a very clear and simple crossroads, and that is where and when you stand by your morals and principles – or you don't. You get deep in the valley of life, which is a very simple place to be, and that, possibly, was the biggest thing that I learnt on that race. Everybody likes to think about how he or she would react in

those circumstances, but I don't think you really know until you get there and I don't necessarily think that because you've made the right decision one time, you'd make it a second time.

So I ventured up on deck, turned the boat around and the fight began. I had to think of it as a fight and screaming at the wind and waves helped strengthen my resolve. Even so, turning the boat into the wind meant that it immediately lay flat on its side. In fact the boat was being knocked down every twenty minutes; it was like being in a perpetual car crash. It was shaken so horribly that the generator was ripped off its engine mounts. If you can imagine picking up a boat and shaking it until the engine falls out that will give you an idea of what it felt like.

The rescue would be broken down into three phases: the first was to try to survive the storm; if we could survive the storm only then would we worry about trying to find the 160 miles. If we could claw them back only then would we worry about trying to find Raphael. This is the process we use with all of our projects. If you have a big challenge or a really big goal, it is very easy to be completely overwhelmed by it – you feel a bit like the proverbial rabbit in the headlights – so we always plan a path with measurable milestones and you just keep chewing off bits of it as you go along. You can change your course at each milestone, just adjusting a little bit.

In the end we did manage to get back and had a successful outcome, thanks in large part to Raphael's own efforts at his end, which meant that, quite amazingly considering the diabolical conditions he was in, he survived. Eventually, after depositing Raphael in Hobart, I managed to finish the race with a great sense of inner peace.

The Vendée is the Everest of sailing and tests everything: your sailing skills, your project management skills and your business skills. There are two distinct challenges: the first is to get to the start line and the second is to get to the finish. Often the first is as hard, if not harder, than the second. The race itself I do because I enjoy it (something one should never lose sight of in life), so when the start gun goes I have a great sense of relief; life suddenly gets really simple, all you have to do is sail around the world. The building blocks of success in any competition are laid down during the pre-event planning and preparation phase. In ocean sailing, preparation is something we take very seriously, for example these days we work with NASA on sleep patterns. We all have a different sleep pattern, not unlike the way we all have different fingerprints. So if a rough, tough hero-type skipper declares that he hasn't slept for the first four days of a race, it begs the question, in my view, what happens on the fifth day? That will be the day he lost the race. It's a lot about resource management. In the case of food we knew we'd need four and a half thousand calories per day in the tropics (and that goes up to six and a half thousand in the Southern Ocean), so we used freeze-dried food that we mixed up ourselves. We vacuum-packed it with a local butcher's machine (that we had borrowed at night when his shop was closed!) and then all of the food was individually separated into twenty-four bags (i.e. a bag for each week which was how long we thought the race would be) and each day's rations numbered from 1 to 120 in total. What this degree of preparation does is to free you up when you are sailing to devote more of your time and focus on boat speed.

However, once you have crossed the finish line, the competition and the result are largely irrelevant because the event – the profound experience of it – far outweighs them and it. A common question I am asked (usually after a talk about the race) is, 'Where did you come?' It's not something that seems very important.

A single-handed sail around the world is basically you with no excuses, and it's my belief that you learn a lot about yourself and perhaps a lot about life. Although the Vendée Globe was the best thing I've ever done, it certainly made me reconsider my life. After the rescue of Raphael, I thought nothing worse could ever happen again; from now on whatever comes along, it can't be worse, I'll survive. And the sun will always come up in the morning. The one thing I've learnt – and you learn as much from your mistakes as your successes – is do what you do to the best of your ability and, if you get the best out of yourself, then there can be nothing more rewarding.

Mind games

THESE DAYS SPORTS PSYCHOLOGY plays an increasingly important part in my work with clients of all ability levels. Actually, psychology isn't the word I'd use in this context, it sounds too formal and academic. No, what I'm talking about is using my range of experiences in sport to try to understand and interpret what's going on in someone's head, and how an individual's thinking and emotional state might be influencing their performance. Then I try to guide and encourage them to a more positive mind state. Perhaps it's the same thing – I'm not sure, but I prefer to call this aspect of coaching 'mind games'.

Mind games, which include improving confidence levels, maintaining motivation, evolving competitive strategy, visualisation techniques and so on, are critical in many sports, and have an important role to play in your approach to general fitness training as well.

One version of mind games most of us will be familiar with happens every twelve months. If you used to play a lot of sport, but are less active now, you may even lack sufficient motivation to get out of your comfy armchair. I call it the 'New Year's Day Gym Syndrome'. Another year has drifted by and you are determined to get out and exercise more, but a few weeks into this brave new active world you start coming up with a growing list of excuses of why you can't make the next session.

Much of this is down to initially setting unrealistic goals and aims. Don't give yourself six weeks before a vacation to lose all the weight you put on in the last twelve months or forty years for that matter! And, if you are hitting your middle years, don't think that motivation is about signing up for the next marathon when you haven't remotely started to get your body into any sort of condition. Setting yourself challenges that are too difficult for your current state of fitness will only overstretch your body too soon. And let's face it, we all have enough pressures in our modern lives without adding any more that we don't really need. See the section on setting your goals on pages 81-82 and have another look at Basic conditioning on pages 90–97, which will give you a broad outline of what you need to be doing and help keep your mind focused so you don't lose interest and let yourself down.

The opposite of setting targets that impose too much pressure is not setting any at all, which is a problem I often see among club athletes. They reach a certain level of performance and then forget to keep looking for new challenges – they're just turning up for the sessions in a perfunctory kind of way. Then they wonder why they're not achieving anything more, why they're on a performance plateau. Whatever your level of sport or intensity of training, from the elite athlete to those of you starting out on a basic conditioning programme, it is

Why are you reading this chapter? Have you lost the will to go back to the gym, lost the will to live? Read on...

really important to come away from every session having learned something new or in a positive mind state about your progress. For example you might say to yourself, 'Last week I gave up on my run at this point' and use it as an incentive to go the extra mile. After twenty-five years of training every day, I still look to gain something from every session, an incremental improvement in my riding technique for example.

Again, if you think you fall into the category of stalled progress, then have another look at the chapter called Where are you now? It's designed to get you over this phase.

Above all, if exercising is not fun any more, it's definitely time to review what you're doing. Fun is whatever you want it to be: it could be running your first 10km race, crossing the finishing line, feeling close to exhaustion, feeling nauseous, but also feeling ten feet tall because of what you have achieved. And remember it might not always be out-and-out fun having to train all of the time, but the buzz it creates in your daily life should carry you through the harder sessions. That's what you've got to remember when the 6am alarm goes off to get you out of bed for that early morning run before work! Get the feelgood factor back, and don't give up.

Before reading this book, you may, in the past, have tried to improve your fitness levels and performance – maybe even sat down and written out some of those lists we talked about earlier in the book, but somehow you just couldn't get your programme going, let alone sustain any sort of momentum. My advice is this: you

need a process to get you on the way. This process starts with Basic conditioning (pages 90–97) and goes right through to preparing for a specific sport or event. Remember everybody always talks good fitness at the beginning of each year; few people actually carry it through. Make a point of being one of the minority who do.

So, mentally throw out all the excuses: why you can't find the time or the inner motivation to get fit, why you somehow can't get started. The only person you're kidding is yourself. And it doesn't matter how much kit you buy, or what fancy new sports toys you flash about – at the end of the day it boils down to some hard work. There, I've said it.

There is no magic formula, no short cut to having a six-pack like Denise Lewis. I firmly believe that there's something special in all of us, untapped potential if you like, but our modern-day lifestyles mean we have become soft. Most of us are not mentally tough – clever yes, but tough, no. I don't like to bang on about it, but there's no doubt that the Marines taught me about tough living and they are the reason why I can't get my head around, or tolerate, sloppy training methods, poor technique, lateness and so on. We only get one shot at life, so it makes sense to learn and adopt the discipline to get the most out of yourself – both physically and mentally.

As a Marine we used to do a fast 10–30km hike with a fully loaded Bergen. At the finish it was a natural reaction to put our hands on our knees and stay bent over to rest and recover. 'Stand up Shrosbree', the PTIs would bark. They

Discipline has been the foundation of my sporting life. It has got me to the point where I can dig deep and know I'll find that bit more and win...

were looking for and instilling self-discipline. The Marines wanted more out of us at every turn and, in time, it meant that even when I felt I'd given absolutely everything, I could dig that bit deeper and find another level of performance. Surprise yourself – you are capable of far more than you think.

The main motivating thought you should keep uppermost in your mind at all times is how great you will feel because you will have got fit for yourself. What I'm trying to tell you, in a roundabout way, is that the bottom line is that it won't be easy – but it will be rewarding. Trust me! Now get your trainers on and get cracking.

There you have it, the proverbial kick up the backside some of you are looking for. You might want to read this little bit from time to time when you are about to settle into the armchair, muttering, 'Forget it, I'll go down the gym tomorrow instead...'

My father is in his mid-70s, suffers from some arthritis and he has had a knee implant. He used to love his cycling (see the picture on page 8) and always enjoyed the outdoors. He called me the other week to say that he was on a Royal Yachting Association Laser sailing course on Rutland Water. I tip my hat to him: he's still getting out there, feeling good, looking for new challenges. So as well as *Inspired* by Bernie Shrosbree, this book should also be called *Inspired* by Charlie Shrosbree.

Mind games for athletes

At a more advanced level, athletes put an incredible amount of pressure on themselves, and react badly whenever they fail to achieve their goals because the pressure is too intense. They beat themselves up over their training programme, frightened of changing the structure, worrying about missing sessions. Just as for the rest of us, there is no short cut to excellence and the work has to be done, but it should be done in the context of an overall aim.

It's all about attitude.

I once took a group of professional mountain bikers for a training session at the Renault F1 Team Human Performance Centre. I suggested they do some training on the Monday. 'We don't train on Mondays', they told me, because they had races on Sunday, so 'obviously' they needed the day after off. And they'd got that fixed in their heads. My view was that with an active recovery programme of massage and stretching, they ought to be straight back out doing some activity on the Monday, although not necessarily in the saddle; maybe swimming or some gym-based light weight training. They had allowed themselves to get stuck in a routine, which was both a mental barrier when it came to considering any changes to their training schedules and, as usual, guaranteed they would hit a performance plateau sooner or later, which in turn would mean general depression and training fatigue.

Some variety, some fresh thinking every few weeks, will help you keep enjoying what you're doing at the competitive level. There are many ways to combine all the ingredients in this book. If you stick to the same diet every day, you'll soon get bored. So mix things up, try to add spice to your exercise. It's all about combining ingredients and spicing up your programme. Think of me as the Jamie Oliver of fitness! Mixing up the training programme can help to avoid the mental staleness that athletes encounter training day in day out, and produce a better result or performance come race day.

Another way that athletes try to get the best out of themselves is by using training camps and training groups to vary what they're doing. If you train with the same bunch of guys or girls the whole time, try getting out on your own from time to time. And away from the head banging and niggling that sticking in the same group

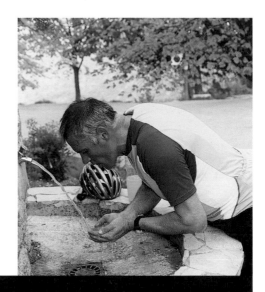

The Col de la Madone

The great Lance Armstrong and I have one thing in common: to test our fitness we both use a fabulous, but incredibly tough, climb in the Maritime Alps. In Lance's case as preparation for the Tour de France, and in mine to examine the conditioning and mental stamina of several F1 drivers.

The Col de la Madone is a climb that starts at close to sea level in the village of Menton, a few miles from the haven of F1 drivers, Monaco, and rises for 927 metres. Lance holds the record of 30 minutes 47 seconds and describes it as the ultimate test. He knows that when he can complete the climb in a time not far off his record, he's ready for the Tour.

At St Agnes, about three quarters of the way up on a somwhat extended route and after forty minutes of hard riding, there is a fountain which Mark Webber, Jenson Button and Ralph

Firman call the prayer stop. Because they pray we'll stop (to refill our water bottles).

Pushing delicate F1 drivers to the edge of their physical limits on an extreme climb might seem an odd way to behave, but picture, if you can, the way the harsh summer heat radiates back from the tarmac and reflects off the white rocks that border the road, the way it saps the riders' strength and plays on their minds. We end up thinking much more about tolerating the heat than the physical effort of the climb itself. But this is what it's all about for me. The cockpit of a racing car is an unimaginably hostile environment, with temperatures often exceeding 50°C. These drivers have to learn to focus one hundred percent on driving the car rather than their massive physical discomfort. So as we climb the Col de la Madone we're training for a purpose.

The fountain at the 'prayer stop' in St Agnes

can create. Conversely, if you are a loner when training, try mixing in with some other athletes from time to time. This will liven up your sessions and test you in different ways to the solo efforts you're used to. When I was training full time for triathlon, I used to train with a top local swim team a couple of times a week, a top class runner called Brent Jones (Brent ran a 2 hour 17 minutes marathon at the age of 20) and for my last (and best) season, with top cyclist Mark Fodden. I didn't do this every day, but enough to test and stretch me mentally and physically on a regular basis. I remember feeling physically sick on the way over to Mark's house to go riding on a Wednesday night: I knew it was going to be a really hard ride of up to 70 hilly miles, and that I would be hanging on for grim death all the way. I hated it so much I actually sort of liked it – if you know what I mean. Every week I would pray for rain so that the session would be called off, but would feel disappointed with myself if I had to miss it. The upshot of this training was that I had my best ever year in triathlon, cycling much faster than I had done in previous years and a lot of that was due to the combination of physical and mental toughness that was created by those evenings of hell with bloody Fodden!

What you can take from this is that sometimes it is good to put yourself in situations where you feel a bit under pressure. You can learn to cope with it gradually – it's what will happen in a race or competition. Don't make the mistake of being too tough on yourself and doing it

all of the time though. This just leads to mental and physical burnout with your best performances left out on the training ground where nobody was there to witness them…

Competition mind games

When the going gets tough … you know the phrase. It may be a cliché, but that doesn't stop it being very true!

People have asked me why I think I thrived in the tough competitions like *Survival of the Fittest*. Competitions that needed a competitor to be superfit, but also endure some pretty extreme environments and still keep it together upstairs, solve problems and race tactically all the way. I think it's largely down to what I would describe as an individual's tolerance to discomfort, and a bit of intelligent thinking under pressure. In the Marines I was sometimes put in situations where I was under a lot of mental stress, often physical stress too, and I had to perform my job perfectly – otherwise, well … you can probably guess that the consequences could be pretty dire. This means that my own 'comfort zones' of putting up with physical discomfort and mental stress are probably a bit more extreme than most other people's. I also think that the biathlon training I did, during which I had to swap from the extreme physical stress of cross-country skiing to the mentally tough concentration of target shooting, gave me an edge too. For the first couple of years I competed in the biathlon, I was too keen to blat off all of my rounds as quickly as possible, to get out of the range and chase down the other guys. Unfortunately, as a result I just spent a lot of time skiing around penalty loops, and after a while the realisation that I was going to have to work on achieving a controlled stillness (not so easy when your heart rate is a high percentage of its maximum) on the shooting range sunk in.

So think about all the performance factors in your sport. Can you apply the old grey matter a bit more effectively to take you up to the next level'?

We are individuals with different personalities, and what motivates you or I on the day will be different, as will how each of us deals with pressure. I've always been the same: I need to nip behind a hedge just before a race, whether it's a world championship or fathers' race at my kids' school. Some athletes need to be alone and to keep quiet; others like to talk their way out of their nervousness. You have to try different ways of approaching your events to see how you respond – it's a very individual thing and it doesn't matter what you do as long as it fills you with the confidence, and develops the mindset you need to perform to your best. You see this in different sports: with the boxers who love to try to belittle and humiliate their opponents in the pre-fight hype or sprinters who psych each other out on the warm-up track. Other athletes might prefer to talk their chances down to take the pressure off their shoulders and pile it onto someone else's. See what works best for you.

When the starting gun goes, if you're of equal physical ability, it's the person with the extra mental strength and the hunger to be a winner who will prevail. The difference between the good and the great performer is often found in the head not in the body – most top athletes will be in really similar physical shape, so it has to be the attitude and tactics that make a difference and a winner.

A great example of a top athlete playing mind games was distance runner Paula Radcliffe when she set a new world record of 2 hours 15 minutes in the 2003 London Marathon. After the race she said that in sections towards the end she was counting up to one hundred over and over. She was doing this to keep focused on the pace and the rhythm she was trying to maintain. There was no threat from other athletes around her to push her on as the second-placed woman was minutes behind, and Paula effectively had the race won. The counting rhythm allowed her to keep her mind on the task in hand rather than thinking about something else to ease the pain, which might have meant her slowing down and not setting a sub 2.16 time. Remember this the next time you're out on a tough session: forget what you might have for tea tonight and get mentally tapped into what you're doing.

And remember David Beckham's total concentration when he took that crucial pressure penalty against Argentina in the 2002 World Cup: he was able to shut out all of the distractions in the stadium, a worldwide television audience of nearly 400 million holding its collective breath, and stay utterly focused, visualising the ball in the back of the net. Live the moment – and come out a winner in the mind games.

Fit to compete *Colin McRae*

Sometimes injury can interrupt the best-planned training programme. But what happens if the injury is actually caused by your sport and is sufficiently serious to be career (or life) threatening? Just how do you overcome the understandable confidence-sapping aftermath and get back out there?

One sportsman who found out the hard way was World Champion rally driver Colin McRae, who experienced a terrifying and potentially fatal crash during the Rally of Corsica in 2000.

Colin and his navigator Nicky Grist were lying fourth overall in their Ford Focus when it left the road after a series of sixth gear bends and ended up in a ravine. "The crash itself was a very straightforward accident which nine times out of ten you would walk away from, but the thing is with any accident if you hit something the wrong way you've got a good chance of injuring yourself and that's what happened. I was unlucky, Nicky walks away without a scratch and I end up in hospital.

"The car went through a wall, turned upside down and hit a tree which did all the damage on my side of the car, then it fell down into the ravine. I suffered a heavy blow when we hit the tree and then we sort of tumbled down the banking.

"After we hit the wall I don't remember a lot about it, but Bernie told me later that I was trapped in the car for 45 minutes. From what I can gather the emergency services had almost given up, reporting to race control, 'We can't get him out'. The other problem was that there was a lot of fuel lying around and obviously they were worried about using cutting machinery and sparking something off. I think they were sitting on the bank having a re-think about what they were going to do and meanwhile I was running out of time. I was in and out of consciousness and it was difficult to breathe because of all the blood, but I was reasonably comfortable as you can be in that situation. Then Bernie ropes down the ravine, pulls the door off the car and gets me out. Cheers mate!

"I was flown to hospital where the X-rays showed that the eye socket was smashed quite badly and my cheekbone was a mess. My surgeon couldn't escape my frustration when I said I wanted to be back in the car in two weeks time. It was painful, but I was walking around and in my mind I felt fine. He was concerned about any lasting effects, 'Obviously, your mind is set on doing this', he said. 'I'll do my job, I'll put it all back where it should be, see how you feel and then you make the decision. All you've got to remember is if you have another heavy impact then I might not be able to fix it again.'

"But I felt you have to get back on it straight away. It was a mind game, a psychological thing. This was an injury that could have potentially killed me or caused lasting damage. When you have serious pain or been that close to something very, very serious you do think about it. I have had massive accidents where the car has been

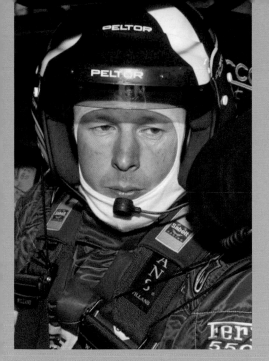

meanwhile is always looking at every possible area to gain performance, and one side of that is the human performance. Conditioning and improved fitness does add to our competitive edge, and probably helped me when I needed it most – hanging upside down in a fuel-leaking, smashed-up rally car.

"Mountain biking was something I had always done and if you are going to stick to a conditioning programme you need to find something you enjoy doing. Running I can't be bothered with; ever seen a happy jogger? Well, that's really unfair on everyone who likes running, but if you don't enjoy jogging you're not going to have that much enthusiasm to keep going so you've got to try to find that thing that you get a reasonable amount of pleasure from and let yourself go at that.

"We're fortunate at this level of motorsport because we can have Bernie work with us, which is a big, big bonus and, because he's generally fitter than us anyway, he can gauge us very well, pulling us along, giving us something to go for. Nicky Grist fell into that trap. He reckoned at one point he was actually getting as fit as Bernie and I sat back and watched as he threw up halfway up the Gorge de Cian climb, trying to keep up with Bernie. He'd always made us feel we were just catching him: he was just being subtle, but he got the balance right. So, with experience and knowledge, planning, preparation and not a little inspiration Bernie gets us to where we want to be. I hope he does the same for you."

destroyed and you walk out of them. You walk away and all you think about is blowing the result; you don't think about the consequences of the accident. In fact, generally you don't do that until you have an injury.

"At this level of motorsport everybody has had accidents, but over the years none of mine have stuck in my mind apart from this one. It made me think about the risks a bit more, but in this work you cannot allow this sort of thing to affect the speed at which you drive. If it does, then it is the time to stop.

"Then it was all about getting fit to drive again with Bernie's help. It's good to have someone who understands what you are going through backing you up all the time, and the thing about Bernie is he really pushes for you for the best physically and, at the same time, mentally.

"To drive a WRC car flat out, or these days a Ferrari 500 Maranello sportscar at Le Mans, you have to have total confidence in the engineers, navigator, everybody in the team. The team

Programme planning

OVER THE LAST 25 YEARS I'VE SEEN training programmes go through almost as many changes in terminology and structural facelifts as celebrity-led diets. And just like nutritional science, the bottom line still remains the same as it ever did: no matter how you tart it up, a programme needs to have enough structure – by which I mean it must employ organised and appropriate levels of training – to push your body into the physical changes you want to see or feel, but crucially also have the flexibility to deal with any 'F' factors that occur (it's an old Marine's phrase – use your imagination for what the F stands for!). Possible F factors might include injury, illness or anything in your day-to-day life that can disrupt the plan.

It would take a whole book and more to explore all the ideas about putting a training programme together; in fact most books and magazines typically get away with describing a few 'case studies' for you to follow. The problem with this approach is that if you've not had a hand in the construction of your own plan, it's all too easy to blame the programme when it goes wrong, doesn't deliver the results you hoped for or you find it simply impossible to stick with.

For most of my life I have had to listen to a sizeable percentage of the people I come into contact with complain that they haven't got the time to really structure, work and commit to a programme. That's

a poor excuse really. It's like anything in life; you know you can make the time for it if you really want to. These days, I need to finish my training by 7.00am much of the time, so I have had to get into a routine where I go to bed early, and am out running or on the water paddling by 5.00am. Then I'll drive for two hours to make my first morning meetings. That's the commitment I give it – I'm 45 and still find training fun and enjoyable. I want to get it across loudly and clearly dear reader that YOU (and only you) have to take responsibility for your day-to-day sessions – while I'll provide the outline structure for you to work with. So pay attention and if necessary go and revisit all those earlier sections in the book to get the ideas and principles fresh in your mind. The most important areas to really understand, so you can safely and effectively construct your own programme, are:

- **Where are you now and where do you want to be?**
- Basic conditioning
- How to progress your training
- The HRM fitness test
- All of the muscle groups/exercises

These sections are like the ingredients list in a cookery book. You don't just throw them all in a bowl and hope that the final dish will be a perfect soufflé, but I reckon that's what the majority of you do in an

Planning a programme doesn't need to be complicated, just well structured.

effort to achieve your goals in sport and fitness. A lot of us go to the gym and because we are only human do things by habit, getting stuck in a rut, plus we usually do things that make us feel good – which is fine to a point. We don't want to go to the gym and participate in an activity that makes us feel miserable, but what we have got to look at is what brings us on in the activity or the sport that we are participating in. Years and years ago I learnt this the hard way, and it's something I would like you to take advantage of here. You must really try to identify your main areas of weakness and have the dedication to work on them as a priority. What I mean is recognise the areas of conditioning in your sport, whether they're on the technical, cardiovascular or the strength side, that are not in balance with your idea of top performance – then spend a lot more time working on these weaknesses, because this is what will bring you on in leaps and bounds. It is the fundamental approach necessary to becoming a good athlete, sportsperson or just basically getting fit for your favourite activity. What I am trying to say here is don't just go and write a recipe of jolly, fun training all the time; what you need to do is start to really identify what is letting you down or is restricting you from performing at a better level. Bear this in mind as you start to plan out what you're going to do.

THE BASIC PHASES OF TRAINING
Right, welcome to Bernie's outline training plan – tried and tested over the last 25 years. I can hold my hands up and say,

The Golden Rules when you start a training programme

- Aim for a minimum of four quality sessions per week for general fitness
- Increase your training volume by 10% per week (much more is risky)
- Do not do hard days back to back
- Try to have no more than two days off in a row
- Prioritise weaknesses but do enough training on your strengths to maintain them
- Be honest with yourself about where you are at – not where you wish you were
- Increase volume before intensity
- Have an aim, even if it's only to maintain the level of fitness you already have
- Learn to understand your own body and know when you need to adapt the programme to include more recovery time or more hard training – this only comes with experience
- Have fun – training should be testing but enjoyable

'Yeah, sometimes I didn't get it quite right for myself', but following a lifetime's experience I am going to give you the facts and describe the methods that have been successful for me, for dozens of world-class elite athletes, sportspeople and a number of ordinary folk with whom

I've worked. The sports science and the fact that I have constantly refined and put into practice what I am about to tell you means that these methods DO WORK. I know they have helped me and a lot of my athletes to achieve some pretty special moments in our sporting careers. The key message to get across is that there is no black and white, no absolute right and wrong, but here I have laid out the methods that will be more likely to succeed than others I have tried. I want you to be able to read this, sit down and think about where you want to go and be armed with enough information and confidence to plan your own programme to get there.

So read on, and then get out there and create some special moments of your own.

BASE TRAINING AND SPECIFIC BASE CONDITIONING PHASES

The Base/Base Conditioning phase is a period of training that will last anywhere between eight and sixteen weeks and will basically help you to create a physical platform to work from for whatever type of activity you are involved in. Simply put, you need to create a robust level of fitness to start with, and that's all about becoming cardiovascularly efficient, and getting or regaining some strength and mobility around your joints and in your major muscle groups. For the serious athlete, the base is about re-creating a foundation to work from after a season or series of events. Obviously if you are in year three of a five-year programme, building up to say a world championship, your base would be at a higher level than

where you started last year. Now that doesn't mean that the base training phase is necessarily just going to be more intense than a year ago – it may just run for a longer period to create more hours of activity and include other conditioning-type exercises to make you stronger in different areas. It varies so much with the individual.

During base conditioning I would encourage you to polish the technical aspects of the activity you're involved in and try some more varied training methods to stimulate your body and mind in different ways. Perhaps you may have to go away and do some lateral thinking and introduce exercises that enhance the basic components of your sport from a new angle (taking the GB rowers cross-country skiing each January for example).

During this phase when you are in the gym strength training, you shouldn't be too worried about how much actual weight you are lifting. Say you have built up to doing some pretty heavy bicep curls and you are performing a sensible amount of repetitions and sets, but actually you are executing these quite poorly mechanically speaking (maybe you are bent over, in other words your arms are strong but your back is weak), you should reduce the load and sort out the technique as well as introducing the right sort of exercises to improve your back and core strength.

This is where the subtleties of Bernie Shrosbree's training methods come into play. I'm trying to get you to think a little more precisely about what you're trying to achieve in the long run, not just the actual

The Shrosbree Perceived Exertion Scale

6. max out
all-out exertion
sprinting flat out. not sustainable for any real length of time

5. severe
race pace
mental and physical battle to sustain pace

4. hard pace
intense training pace
requires commitment and concentration to sustain intensity

3. steady pace
relatively comfortable aerobic training pace
the athlete perceives that work starts at this intensity.
mentally and physically in control

2. easy pace
very comfortable
moderate warm-up pace. no perceived mental
or physical pressure

1. light pace
easy warm-up/recovery
very gentle activity

moment, not just the particular exercise. I'm trying to get you to work in a way so that everything is done properly to build for the future. If everything *is* done properly it will take you to greater heights when you move into your quality phase; the phase when you won't have to worry about whether you are executing an exercise or your sport efficiently because the good habits will already be formed.

Beginners and novice athletes

Remember this phrase in this phase: **Longer, Lower, Regular** (LLR). As a total beginner you can start with the heart rate fitness test on page 87 and start logging daily activity at Levels 2 and 3 on the Shrosbree Perceived Exertion Scale (previous page). To progress during this stage you should be upping the amount of time you're training (the overall volume) – not the intensity. There's nothing wrong with exercising for only a few minutes a day at first, so don't let yourself be put off by other people's locker room stories of mega workouts or the sports stars they've been training with. In my experience those that talk a good workout rarely live up to it in real life. Upping the volume by about 10% per week is a pretty good guideline; sufficient to stress the body without breaking it down. Try to keep this stage going for at least twelve weeks. Sketch out a plan for the next 7–10 days or so and try it out (see pages 252–253 for a guide to a 'typical training week').

Remember that 7-day plans don't have to be the only way of organising your training just because your working week revolves around it. OK, so with this

approach you know more or less what you are doing Monday through to Sunday, but the danger is that not only your life, but your training becomes too set in routine – which stops a lot of people progressing. It was interesting working with the GB Rowing Team during the winter when we were up at altitude in St Moritz. They were on a two and a half day cycle for that particular period; that is two and half days of intense training with a half-day's rest on the third day, repeated three times consecutively. Then they would have a full day's rest, followed by another three cycles of two and half day's intense training and so on. If you asked the guys what they were doing 'next Sunday' they would not know, but if you asked about 'the next half day' they would know straightaway. It kept them focused on the next 48 hours so that they didn't get lost in a psychologically tough 7-day plan.

When I was training for triathlon I would work on a 10-day cycle in the base phase with three lots of ten days, with a day's rest interspersed between each 10-day period. The first two 10-day spells would be filled right up with activity and the third 10-day training spell would be very hard for the first four days and then I would back right off to help the body recover. Maybe you can do something similar, in other words build the volume up over a period of so many days and then make sure you include a recovery phase – something often neglected but vitally important in the long run.

As your body adapts to the training you can gradually apply the 10% rule to increase the volume and you're under way! In essence, this phase is all about growing the nerve pathways to wake up muscle fibres that haven't seen much action for a while and getting your mind and lifestyle used to a regular dose of training. Despite what I've said about 10-day plans and so on, don't be afraid to give yourself a couple or three days of rest per week at first, but try not to have two days off in a row if it can be helped.

Club athletes

For those of you who have already been training at club level or thereabouts and maybe competing from time to time, ask yourself when was the last time that you went back to basics and did three months of steady, Level 2–4 training, to work on pure techniques and body mechanics. For a runner this would be the winter phase, emphasising, long steady runs if your main targets are in the summer track season or, for a swimmer, the main emphasis would be on technical excellence and land training without worrying about being a slave to the ticking clock on the poolside. If it's been more than a year I would seriously recommend factoring in some base work as soon as possible if you want to move your performance level on next season.

Summary of base training

In summary, when you are planning this phase it ideally needs to be eight to sixteen weeks long, emphasising steady state training at exertion Levels 2–4 (2 is more appropriate for total beginners, 3 and occasionally 4 for more experienced

athletes) and some total body conditioning work in the gym. Make sure you review and record your sessions each week (I've included both a weekly training plan and an annual activity log on the inside back cover). The idea should be to start seeing and feeling improvements in efficiency over three to four weeks, and if you're doing resistance work the DOMS (see page 92) should have been and gone completely by week four. Plan a few days in advance, aiming for a few small targets on the way, but don't put pressure on yourself or really test your limits, yet – stay out of the red. The time for that will come later on I can assure you! In this base phase it is best to get as much variety as possible into the sessions, so do some light resistance work with weights and a variety of aerobic activities. My personal favourites, if you want the ultimate combination of sports, would be Concept 2 rowing, indoor or outdoor cross-country skiing (kinder on the knees than a treadmill or jogging) and some resistance gym work with exercises such as the six compound lifts (pages 114–125). But the most important thing is that you can find out what suits you best by experimenting and trying things out for yourself. Bear in mind that there has to be some organisation, but even at the top end of sport, athletes and coaches are pursuing effective training with a degree of trial and error. Some solid basics are adhered to, but the limits are only tested by trying something new. And, frankly, if you're trying out various programmes (and occasionally producing a few errors) then at least you are out training instead of just thinking about it with your backside on the sofa!

Specific base conditioning

If you're a really serious athlete looking to achieve top-end competitive results in your sport then the Base phase will also need to run into a Base Conditioning phase. This is an extended low-intensity period of training but it incorporates much more sports-specific training. For example, as a cyclist you might be doing a lot of cross-country skiing as base work but after a period of this you will have to shift more emphasis onto cycling itself to condition your body precisely for the task at which you want to excel.

Maintenance base training

By the way, I've said allow eight to sixteen weeks for this Base phase, but for some of you this is the start of the rest of your life! Even without burning competitive ambitions or serious physical challenges on your agenda, you will be well on the way to a new level of fitness that will need maintaining through regular topping up – to keep you in great shape for your everyday life. Of course if you should get the urge to take part in the local 10km fun run or even to row the Atlantic, your higher level of base fitness will make you more than ready to step up the training and make it happen, whatever it is, more quickly and with far fewer tears than anyone starting out from zero.

Maintenance training is based on what the first weeks taught you. By now you will have discovered the things you enjoy, are good at and want to keep on doing. These activities and sessions will form the basis of your regular training, but remember to spice it up now and again with a few of those tougher sessions that you're not so keen on. There's nothing wrong with some routine and set patterns in training, but as I've said before, challenging yourself by varying your activities and doing the workouts you're not so keen on is going to be really important in the long run – so you don't get stale and lose motivation over time. Remember: the truth is it pays to have a goal even if it's only to hold onto what you've got.

THE QUALITY PHASE

The Quality phase is a more intensive form of training for those of you who take your sport a lot more seriously or compete actively. If you're contemplating this type of training, you will be in possession of a real desire to achieve your own optimum performance in whatever is your chosen activity or you will have a specific event, such as the regional half marathon, that you see as a challenge and want to properly prepare for. Think of the process like this: you don't just suddenly jump into the Quality phase from the Base Conditioning phase overnight – it's a transitional process where the training becomes increasingly more sports-specific (i.e. you cut back on the general training and move to a situation where you do, almost exclusively, conditioning for your own sport); the intensity level creeps up and, to a certain extent, the volume is reduced to enable you to cope with the rising tempo. In this phase recovery is all-important because you're shocking the body more than with the relatively easy Base workouts. A great example of what I'm talking about would be a runner's fartlek sessions – often used

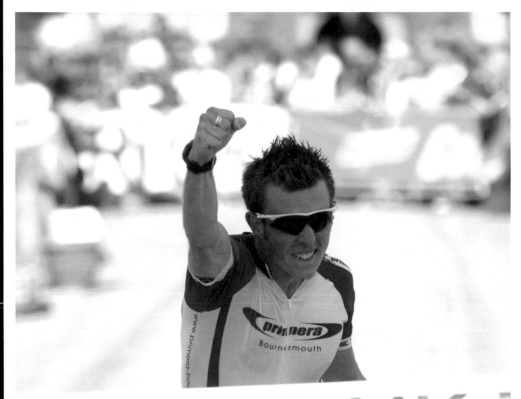

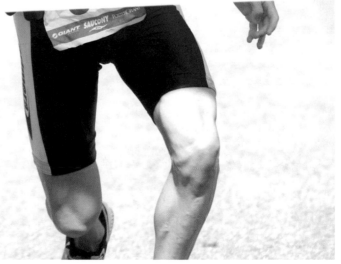

When it all comes together

Specific resistance training

Once you've had a good Base Conditioning phase and you are transitioning into your Quality phase, then what you can do is introduce a more advanced type of overload through sports-specific resistance work – to create greater strength in the muscle fibres, and to build up your tolerance of more intense cardiovascular-type activity.

This resistance overload is usually applied by strength-based interval training, for example sprints on a bike in a big gear for cyclists or uphill running for the athletes out there and, for the rowers, 200-500m bursts on the indoor rower with the damper set to a high level of resistance. It is important to remember that you need to retain a structure in your training when including these types of sessions; you don't just go and row 500m as hard as you can, as many times as you can until you fall off. You should set yourself properly thought-out goals. It's no good saying I am going to do 10 x 500m and after

four reps you can't do another one because the overload has been too high. Gaining an understanding and insight into how you go about doing interval training is key. With running you would start off with only six to eight hill reps of about a minute at a moderate to hard intensity. On the bike you might go for four or five, 5-minute hard spins on the turbo trainer (indoor cycle trainer) in a large gear with relatively low pedal rpm. In the gym (if you're training for very specific lifting strength) you might only do three to six reps of severe overload using heavy weights and only three sets with long recovery intervals.

A note of caution: properly managed specific resistance training can take you to the next level in your performance, but it needs to be built up over a long time, possibly several seasons. If you are not careful and get carried away with too much too soon this type of overload can be your biggest downfall – frankly speaking, it can actually trash you.

during this phase. Fartlek is a Swedish term which means 'speed play' and involves running one of your usual routes, not at a consistent pace but throwing in sections of fast running and sections of jogging recovery. The idea is to gradually increase the length of the fast sections and reduce the jogging until you're basically running the whole route fast. It's a way of progressively

overloading the body with intensive work and that is basically the theme of this phase. It's difficult to generalise, but this phase should be an absolute minimum of four weeks to make any meaningful progress without risking overloading too quickly, but might be as long as three to four months for an endurance athlete with only one main target for the season.

Using competition in this phase

A lot of top athletes will use actual races or competitions within their quality phase of training as a guide to their current form and as ultra-specific workouts in their own right. They won't try to compete at their absolute best in this phase; it simply isn't possible with the relatively high volume of the training, but the events help with things such as practising strategies or tactics, trying new nutritional ideas or equipment and getting that all-important adrenalin rush which only true competition can supply. It is never really a good idea, in my view, to step up to your biggest competitive event of the year with no racing at all under your belt – otherwise it can all come as a bit of a mental and physical shock to the system.

As far as intensity goes you will be moving up from working at Levels 2 and 3 nearly all the time to predominantly Levels 3, 4 with 5 and possibly even a small bit of 6 from time to time. The greatest gains made in this phase come from finding the optimum balance between intensity and volume and that will be determined by the event you wish to do and your level of fitness as you enter this phase. For example, a marathon runner aiming to get under three hours will consider his or her Level 5 activity to be running intervals at 5km race pace or thereabouts on top of a pretty high mileage regime to toughen the legs up for the race itself. A 1500m runner by contrast will not be doing the high marathon-type mileage in this phase, but will instead be focusing on 200, 400 and 800m reps and hill runs as the key intensive sessions to develop the speed

and strength necessary to run 3 1/2 laps of the track virtually flat out. Basically, the 1500m runner will be training generally at a faster pace but covering much less mileage than the marathon runner.

Now please note: it is during this phase that it can all go horribly wrong if you don't manage it correctly. It's about staying on the right side of the divide between the overload the body needs to progress in the training phase and the danger of overtraining. There is in fact only a relatively small difference between optimal overload and overtraining – it's the easiest thing in the world after a great Base/Base Conditioning phase to be in such good shape that you want to go out and train harder and harder to test your new-found abilities. You get these great feelings of invincibility as you fill up the training log with more and more intensive sessions until 'bang' the wheels come off – a torn muscle, a loss of form or plain old fatigue. Group training at this stage is the ultimate nightmare for most club athletes who love to test each other out during every session. I've been there myself on occasions, but don't be tempted to go down this route – not least if you're one of those people who likes to hang back and then sprint the last interval of a set (when the injury might result from a training partner giving you a good kicking for not pacing the session properly!). It is where the classic (and all too true) phrase 'I left my best race out on the training ground' comes from. By all means train with your club or team-mates but don't get sucked into competing when you should be training.

In my early triathlon career, after a good winter's base, I strayed into the red zone a few too many times during the quality phase and found my season ending prematurely. It wasn't until 1989 that I got my triathlon training spot-on – with a gradual build-up in the quality phase after a strong winter base, which enabled me to hold my race form (see the next section) for a whole season and win the British Series, with wins in the first five of the eight rounds.

One key fact to remember is that as you leave this phase and enter the Top Race Form period, you will have taken your basic fitness and strength to its maximum levels. From now on you can't expect to make up lost miles or increase your engine's capacity – the only thing left is sharpening and recovery to bring out your best performance.

Top race form and tapering phase

This phase will last anywhere from about two to four weeks for an athlete preparing solely for one main event to a maximum of a whole season if the goal is to peak for a full series of races or games over the course of a year. The idea of this phase is to maximise the gains made in the previous phases with stimulating but not destructive training. In the quality period you were training hard and frequently, breaking down the body to force it to adapt and build. The top race form and tapering phase is not destructive – its purpose is to enhance recovery, increase energy stores and sharpen you up to perform at your very best.

For an athlete looking at one major peak in the season, the top race form and tapering phase will usually start between two and four weeks ahead of the main event. What you are trying to achieve is to reduce training volume gradually while maintaining elements of intensity at or slightly above race pace. This gets the nerve pathways and muscles used to operating at the speeds needed without putting loads of unnecessary stress on the body as a whole. Ideally, you will find yourself feeling a bit twitchy and restless as the race or big game approaches because your body is used to being fatigued by your training and now is full of energy ready to burn. If you are undertaking an endurance-based event, you will need to eat a bit more than usual in the last few days leading up to the event (no, that's not an excuse to get the pork pies in – healthy carbohydrates are what you need) and drink plenty of water to stay adequately hydrated. You can think of it as the calm before the storm and use the extra time to visualise the event. Check that you are fully organised and try to keep off your feet and rest up (of course your other half may have you painting the windows or something with all your extra free time, but try to resist this temptation!). Sleep is also an interesting aspect of your event preparation to consider as the big day approaches. If you've been training really hard for a while and are used to falling asleep as soon as your head hits the pillow, it might feel a bit odd to find yourself lying awake at night. Don't worry – as long as you are getting a sensible amount of shut-eye you'll be fine on race day even if you don't sleep well the actual

Erratic/guilt training

A word of warning about erratic or guilt training; regularity and consistency are the keys to a successful outcome in any plan. Everyone likes to feel that they are making progress and everyone enjoys being up for a challenge, but too many people train erratically. Even though you've not been to the gym for a few days or even a couple of weeks, you will have a day when you are feeling good, so you decide to really go for it. And sometimes you can pull off a good training session, but what you've got to look at is whether, when you wake up the next day, you can repeat another good quality training session and repeat it the day after that.

If you go flat out in the gym sporadically, yes you are physically working and taxing the body and it does give you a sort of result in improving your performance – certainly over doing nothing – but the danger is that you are straying into the territory of possible injury and disillusionment. It will be the last

couple of kilometres straining on the rowing machine or the last few hundred metres on the treadmill running flat out that will cause microtears in your muscle fibres, a torn hamstring or will give you a knee or back problem. And it's the same with lifting the weights aggressively or in an out-of-control manner. Getting injured could end up putting you off your training for good. Believe me, I've seen it far too many times.

At the risk of repeating myself, you need to be disciplined. Say to yourself, 'Right I've been away from here for three weeks, what do I want to achieve from this?' The key thing is to make sure that you can work out for a regular amount of time four or five times a week, and for a good couple of months – that will get you back into it. And make sure the intensities are right for the programme; then you will reap the benefits a few weeks down the road rather than feel demoralised because you've overdone it early on and seem to be going backwards.

night before – it's the week or so leading up to the event that's important.

For the week-in-week-out athlete (racing in a series or on a competitive circuit) or the serious sportsperson (i.e. those of you who play a team sport like football), the top race form period is very different. You can't afford to be tapering for four months or however long the season lasts because

eventually your fitness will simply slope off and you'll be left well off the pace. In this situation you have to pick out the key races or matches and taper more precisely for them, competing while in training mode through some of the lesser races or games to maintain fitness. The art of holding race form for a whole season takes years of training to really master and is the Holy

Grail for top international athletes. Time and time again you see the more experienced athletes performing at the top of their form from day one to the end of a long season, whereas the less experienced competitors do well initially, but their performances often decline as the season reaches its midway point and beyond. With races or events every weekend, and some midweek competitions too, top athletes will only train at a relatively easy pace between close competitions – sleeping and eating well to recover. For endurance sports it's important to keep some decent high volume training in between events from time to time, but this should be at nice easy Levels 2 and 3, so that it doesn't become destructive.

The team sport players among you will also have to factor in a maintenance programme for dealing with the inevitable knocks and strains associated with impact sports. They will consist of rehabilitation time, agility and speed sessions as well as some long steady training to keep the aerobic engine well maintained and fuelled. It all adds up to a pretty full week in the season and makes the next phase massively important if you want a decent long-term sporting career.

RECOVERY PHASE

Without doubt the Recovery phase is the most neglected phase for a lot of keen athletes and sportspeople. You must allow for some mental and physical recuperation after a big race, game or season. Otherwise your next pre-season Base phase will be badly compromised, and it will all have a negative impact on the forthcoming season.

There is always a temptation to start back training that bit earlier, that bit keener than everyone else by cutting recovery time short – WRONG! You've convinced yourself that by doing so you'll be getting ahead of the game, but it nearly always ends in you peaking too early and a disappointing season that tails off at the end. All you'll really be left with is a lot of excuses for why it didn't happen for you.

So what is recovery? It can be a de-training phase when you are doing a small amount of low impact, light intensity, low volume training with plenty of days off, right through to a two to four week layoff – it's quite an individual thing. I've never been someone who could take a complete rest or entirely absent myself from my sport or training for any length of time – I usually find an enjoyable alternative activity to do. Glenn Cook (the top British triathlete in the 1980s and 1990s), on the other hand, always had a three-week pig-out at the end of the season, and it seemed to work for him – zero training and eating everything he didn't allow himself during the summer was his way of letting go. Decide for yourself how you want to handle it, but whatever you do make sure you plan ahead and get in a good recovery period.

Don't be unduly concerned or put off if you restart your base training a bit below par compared with some of your competitors because you've had a longer (and, therefore, more effective) recovery time – trust me, it will develop into a psychological advantage in the months ahead as you start to turn on the training and they wonder what's going on as you gradually sneak up on them.

A typical training plan for a fitness club member

I often get asked to describe a typical training plan for the non-professional athlete – the guy or girl with an underused gym membership burning a hole in their wallet, the go-get-fitters as I call them. It's very hard to provide an all-inclusive answer because it's such an individual thing, but what it boils down to is asking yourself two simple questions: 'Why do I want to do this and how much commitment and time am I prepared to give it?' In answer to the first part of the question, is it because you want to be fitter, look better or have you set yourself some sort of physical challenge that you know you must prepare for?

But perhaps the more important part of your answer (which must be honest and then stuck to) is the second one. What is the level of commitment you can and are prepared to give to your programme? To be clear about this, any serious training plan designed to deliver measurable improvements in your base levels of fitness is going to require four or more well-planned sessions per week. Sorry, but there really are no quick fixes when it comes to conditioning, whatever other magazines and fitness videos tell you. You're going to have to work honestly at a plan like the one on the right for five to six weeks MINIMUM – before you start seeing and feeling any major changes. So do not be put off if you're not toned and athletic after session 2. Stick with it though and the improvements and rewards will start to become self-evident – and then you'll be hooked.

What these sessions need to do is basically get your engine going and, in the context of the training plan, they fall into the Base phase, which should run for a lengthy period of time.

Here is the outline:
Day one, first session: A cardiovascular session, which could be a 20 to 60 minute mixture of everything from the bike, the rowing machine or the treadmill. It could, for example, be a warm-up on the rower followed by an aerobics class. And it's all done at Level 2 to 3 on the Shrosbree Perceived Exertion Scale (page 241)

Day two: no training – rest day

Day three, second session: An all-over strength conditioning workout, which basically means going around the resistance machines. You would probably do a 10-15 minute warm-up – on a bike or stepper for example – some light mobility exercises and then spend 45 minutes or so doing quality conditioning exercises to strengthen the muscles. This means moderate weights and two or three sets of 10+ repetitions. After a couple of these sessions you'll know areas that you are not so good at, or, if you have access to a good personal trainer or instructor at your club, he or she should be able to guide you towards the areas you need to work on – then just do it! But don't just keep doing the things you feel comfortable with.

Day four: no training – rest day

Day five, third session: Another cardiovascular session, but this time it could

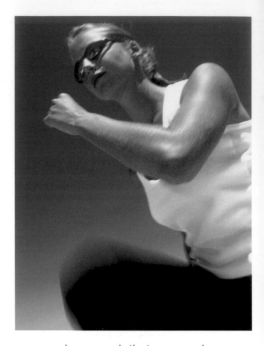

be more geared to your specific sport or to your goal or challenge. So if you were planning to take part in an endurance charity bike ride for example, you would obviously spend more time on the bike in the gym during this session – a spin class followed by a steady ride by yourself, maybe. The idea in this session is to concentrate on the real specifics of your goal and prepare your body for it in a very targeted way. The aimed intensity will be at around Level 3 for the whole of this session.

Day six: no training – rest day

Day seven, fourth session: A totally open and free choice session. This could be an outdoor adventure if you have the time and want to get out in the environment. Literally anything from a hike in the hills to a swim in the sea if your goals are quite general, through to a long run if you've opted to try the local 10km fun run. Equally it could be a second strength-type session back in the gym if you think that's what you need, or a core stability workout and some yoga if your flexibility needs attention. Use this day to really spice up the training plan and enjoy yourself. That way you'll be more motivated for the other sessions and challenge yourself in more varied ways.

OK, that's given you an outline of what I would suggest for somebody who says, 'Look, I've just come back into training and I can commit to four sessions a week.' I've made sure there are two cardiovascular sessions in there, an all-round conditioning-type programme and

one session a week that you can keep entirely flexible – which might mean it is more outdoor-oriented, sports-specific, strength work, core stability work or even working on flexibility. It could just be a general fun session where you turn up and fancy having a go at everything without any stress. Over the weeks the idea is to increase the length of time you are spending in each session, to increase the training stress and stimulate improvement. Hey, congratulations you are in training!

The only thing left to say is don't be too naïve and treat this as an exact blueprint for guaranteed success; make sure you adapt the ideas here for your own programme and accommodate your own strengths, weaknesses and aims. It's something designed to get you up and mobile four times a week. And believe me, if you've not been doing much for a few years, four sessions a week will have a massive and positive impact on your health and quality of life – if you're prepared to stick with it.

Index

A

abdominals 211
aerobic and anaerobic training 98–9
anaerobic threshold 98–9
Annapurna Triathlon Challenge 18
annual activity log *see* inside back cover
arms **164–75**
  bench dips 173
  biceps curl 166
  combination exercises 174–5
  concentration curl 168
  hammer curl 168
  machine dips 172
  reverse curl 169
  triceps extension and kickback 170
  wrist exercises 175
Lance Armstrong 97, 233

B

back *see* upper back; trunk and lower back
back extension (core stability) 112
base training 240
basic conditioning 75, **90–103**
basic phases of training **239–240**, 251
Oli Beckingsale 95, 96, 104
bench dips 173
bench press 122–3
Benetton F1 team 20
biathlon 12, 22, 25
biceps 164–5, 166–9
biceps curl 166
Andy Blow 96
Neil Bowman 12, 17, 28, 96
breaststroke 56
breathing cycle (swimming) 58–9
Robin Brew 55, **60–61**, 66
buoyancy 57
Jenson Button 105, 113, 233

buying a bike 51–53

C

cable crossovers 162
cable crunch with twist 181
cadence 33
calf raises 196
calves 216
Canadian canoeing 67
canoeing *see also* kayaking 9, 16
cardiovascular 77
  drift 87
  efficiency 42, 240
  equipment in the gym 100, 103
chest **154–63**
  cable crossovers 162
  chest press 158
  flys 160
  press-ups 156
chest heave 152
Col de la Madone 233
competition in the quality phase 246
compound exercises **114–25**, 243
  bench press 122–3
  deadlift 116–17
  incline bench press 159
  push press or jerk 124–5
  squat 118 19
  squat and curl 120–21
concentration curl 168
Concept2 *see* indoor rower
Conquer the Arctic 19–20
cool down *see* warm-up
core stability 76, **104–13**, 163
  back extension 112
  F1 driver 113
  kneeling position 109
  pendulum roll 111
  roll-out & press-up 110
  superman 111

  supine bridge position 108
James Cracknell **4–5**, 68, 71, **72–3**
cradle curl 179
crawl *see* frontcrawl
cross-country ski machine 79
cross-country skiing 4, 25, **74–9**, 91, 133, 220, 243
  benefits of 76
  techniques 76–7
cycling **42–53**
  equipment set-up 47
  safety and equipment 46
  suspension, balance and braking 49–51
  what to wear 46

D

deadlift 116–17
deltoids 129, 132
distance running technique 33
diving 15
DOMS 92, 243
dumbbell raises 132

E

endurance running 29
environment 9, 42, 62, 68, **218–29**
erratic/guilt training 249

F

F1 driver (core stability) 113
fast twitch muscle fibres 35
fitness goals *see* goals and goal setting
fitness levels *see* self-analysis
flys 160
forearms 211
frontcrawl 56, 60
functional training *see* core stability

G

gear ratios in cycling 48–9

goals and goal setting 83

golden rules 239

good morning (exercise) 189

Pete Goss 16, **225–29**

Rick Grice 11, 12, 63

group training 31–2, 233, 247

guilt training *see* erratic training

H

hammer curl 168

hamstrings 28, 214

Paul Hart 39

heart rate 38

heart rate fitness test 87–8, 94

heart rate monitors 84, **86–9**

heart rate training zones 88

hexagonal jumps 200

Hinault formula (cycling) 47

hip flexors and extensions 185

hip stretch 213

hurdle jumps 201

hyperextension 47

hypoxic training 58

I

ice skating 79

incline bench press 159

indoor rower 69, **70–1**, 72–3, 243

injury 16, 29, 32, 39, 55, 91, 107, 249

J

jogging 27

jumps

hexagon 200

hurdle 201

lateral 202

K

K1 and K2 23, 64–5

kayaking *see also* canoeing 23, 25,
62-7, 104–5, 222

Canadian canoeing 67

kayak comparison chart 66

sea/coastal and expedition paddling 66

white water racing 66, 222

knee lift (running) 34

kneeling position (core stability) 109

L

lat pull-down 146

lateral jumps 202

latissimus dorsi (lats) 138

legs **190–203**

calf raises 196

hexagonal jumps 200

hurdle jumps 201

lateral jumps 202

lunges 194–5

machine exercises 198

squat jumps 192

step-ups 193

Long Term Athlete Plan 55

Longer, Lower, Regular 37, 84, 97,
98, 242

lower back *see* trunk and lower back

lunges 194–5

Arthur Lydiard 29, 32, 91

M

machine dips 172

machine exercises (legs) 198

maintenance base training 244

maximum heart rate 86

Colin McRae 20, 23, 45, **236–37**

medicine ball 183, 186–87

mind games **230–31**

mountain biking 43–4

muscle groups **127–203**

N

neck 136, 208

shoulder shrugs 137

upright row 136

O

oblique crunch 180

oblique stretch 212

ocean swimming 59

off-road running 32–3

overload training 247

overtraining 85, 86, 247

oxygen 98

P

pectorals 131

pendulum roll (core stability) 111

personal trainers 92

PNF (Proprioceptive Neuromuscular
Facilitation) 217

press-ups 156

Prodrive 20

progression in your training **38–41**

pull-ups 148

push press or jerk 124–5

Q

quadriceps 28, 190, 216

quality phase 244

R

rally of Corsica 46

recovery phase **250**

Renault F1 Team 20, 93, 232

reverse curl (arms) 169

reverse curl (trunk) 184

reverse lateral raise 151

David Richards 20

roll-out and press-up (core stability)110
rollerblading 78
rotator cuff rotation 134
rowing **68–73**, 77
Royal Marines 6, 12, 16, 31, 62, 74, 225
running **25–41**
competitive 30–33
endurance 29–30
equipment 37
jogging 27–9
sprinting 35

S
Carlos Oaina 20
seated row 140
self-analysis (fitness levels) 80–81
shoulders **128–37**, 209
dumbbell raises 132
rotator cuff rotation 134
shoulder press 130
shoulder shrugs 137
upright row 136
Charlie Shrosbree 8, 232
Shrosbree perceived
  exertion scale *see* inside front cover
  29, 79, **241**
side bend 182
single-arm row 143
skiing *see* cross-country skiing
slalom (kayaking) 65
souplesse 43, 49, 97
Special Boat
  Services (SBS) 6, 14, 67, 220
specific base conditioning 244
specific resistance training 246
sprinting 35
squat 118–19
squat and curl 120–21
squat jumps 192
stability balls *see* Swiss balls

steady-paced training 29
steady state training **98**, 100, 103
step machine 102–3
step-ups 28, 193
stomach muscles *see* abdominals
stretching *see also* warm-up
forearms and abdominals 211
hips 213
'hugging the mother-in-law' 210
lower back and hamstring 214
neck and shoulders 208–9
PNF (Proprioceptive
Neuromuscular Facilitation) 217
quadriceps and calves 215, 17
trunk and obliques 212
upper back, shoulder and upper
arms 210
stride length 33
Superman (core stability) 111
supine bridge position 108
Survival of the Fittest 6, 16–17, 33,
  66, 222, 233
swimming **54–61**, 96
efficiency 57
Swiss balls **104–13**, 184, 186,
  204–16
height chart 108
Symond's Yat 62

T
tapering phase *see* top race form
T-bar row 144
Mike Tindall 35
top race form phase **248**
track (running) 30
treadmill 37, 79, 93, 94, **100–102**
triathlon 18–19, 44, 242, 248
triceps extension and kickback 170
trunk and lower back **176–89**, 212, 214
advanced trunk work 186

cable crunch with twist 181
cradle curl 179
good morning 189
hip flexors and extensions 185
oblique crunch 180
reverse curl 184
side bend 182
trunk curl 178
turnover (leg speed) 33
typical training plan **251–52**

U
upper back **138–53**
chest heave 142
lat pull-down 146
pull-ups 148
reverse lateral raise 151
seated row 140
single-arm row 143
T-bar row 144
upright row 136

V
Vendée Globe 226–29
VO₂ max 81

W
walking 32, **35-7**, 84, 93
warm-up 55, **204–17**
waxing (cross-country skiing) 77
Mark Webber 4, 113, 233
weekly training plan *see* inside back
  cover
weight loss 82–3
weight rack 137
white water racing (kayaking) 66
wrist exercises 175

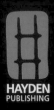

HAYDEN
PUBLISHING

Publisher: Jonathan Hayden
Publishing consultant: Philip Dodd
Associate writer: Andy Blow
Design: Derek Slatter, Fiona Andreanelli and Caz Jones
Illustrations: Alan Fraser (care of Pennant inc.
www.pennantinc.co.uk)

First published in the United Kingdom
by Hayden Publishing
1 2 3 4 5 6 7 8 9 10

Design and layout © Hayden Publishing 2004
Text © Bernie Shrosbree and Hayden Publishing 2004

The right of Bernie Shrosbree to be identified as the author
of this work has been asserted by him in accordance with
the Copyright, Designs and Patents Act 1988.

A CIP catalogue record for this book can be obtained from
the British Library.

Colour reproduced by PDQ Digital Media Solutions Ltd,
Bungay, United Kingdom.

Printed and bound in Italy by Printer Trento.

ISBN 1 90363 504 7

Hayden Publishing
42–44 Dolben Street
London
SE1 0UQ

Bernie's website: www.bernieshrosbree.com

Acknowledgments

The publishers would particularly like to thank
the following who gave generously of their
expertise and time, and without whose help
this book would have been a poorer thing:
Andy Blow whose diligence and discipline
got us there in the end; Mark Webber, star
model and all-round good guy; Ralph Firman
for helping the publisher up and down the
mountain; Colin McRae who didn't mind
interrupting a busy testing session for Le
Mans; Pete Goss for his words and advice;
James Cracknell, always a gentleman; The
GB Rowing Team; The Renault F1 Team; Ian
Hughes at SCOTT Sports Ltd; The Circle
Health Club, especially Sarah Ogole.

Images
© Jonathan Hayden/Hayden Publishing Ltd: 1, 6(t), 10, 20, 23,
24, 26(t), 34, 36, 38(t), 40, 42(t), 43, 58, 62, 63, 67, 68(t), 68, 69,
74(t), 77, 80, 82, 90(t), 90, 97, 99, 114(t), 127, 138(t), 147, 176(t),
217, 221, 230(t), 233, 238(t)
© **Hayden Publishing Ltd photographed by Jonny Ring:** 1 (3rd
from l), 79, 87, 101, 103, 105–113, 116–125, 130–137, 140–146,
148–153, 156–163, 166–175, 178–189, 192–203, 208–216
© **gettyimages:** photographed by Clive Mason; 1 (2nd from l), 45,
204(t), 206 and photographed by Mark Thompson; 22, 57
© **Action Images:** 1(r) 54(t), 55, 127(t), 128, 138, 154(t), 154,
164(t), 190(t), 190, 197, 218(t), 223, 224, 252

In addition the publishers would like to thank the following for their
kind permission to reproduce their photographs: Ford Motorsport:
1(l), 65; James Cracknell: 5, 72, 73, 75; The Renault F1 Team/LAT:
7, 21, 27, 30, 31, 44, 65; SCOTT Sports Ltd: 50, 53, 95, 218;
Concept2: 70–71; Polar Heart Rate Monitors: 88–89; © LAT: 237;
Rick Tomlinson/Rick Tomlinson Photography: 223;
Tim Moxey/digitaltriathlon.com: 245; and the author: 8, 10, 13–19,
26–28, 42, 54, 76, 78.

l = left, r = right, t = top